EYE-DEA
TO
IMPACT

BRAD HALL, PHD

EYE-DEA TO IMPACT

A MODERN BLUEPRINT FOR INVESTIGATOR-INITIATED TRIALS

Numberless
PRESS

info@numberlesspress.com

ISBN: 978-1-0697178-1-8 (paperback)
ISBN: 978-1-0697178-2-5 (ebook)
ISBN: 978-1-0697178-0-1 (hardcover)
ISBN: 978-1-0697178-3-2 (special edition hardcover)

Ordering Information:
Special discounts are available on quantity purchases by corporations, associations, and others. For details, contact info@numberlesspress.com

Publisher's Cataloging-in-Publication Data
Names: Hall, Brad, 1987- .
Title: Eye-dea to impact : a modern blueprint for investigator-initiated trials / Brad Hall, PhD.
Description: [Canada] : Numberless Press, 2025. | Summary: Guides independent ophthalmology and optometry clinics in designing, launching, and completing investigator-initiated trials without disrupting their busy practices. Demystifies the research process and empowers practitioners to turn ideas into real-world impact.
Identifiers: ISBN 9781069717832 (special edition hardcover) | ISBN 9781069717801 (hardcover) | ISBN 9781069717818 (pbk.) | ISBN 9781069717825 (ebook)
Subjects: LCSH: Ophthalmology – Research. | Optometry – Research. | Clinical medicine – Research. | BISAC: MEDICAL / Ophthalmology. | MEDICAL / Optometry. | MEDICAL / Research.
Classification: LCC RE58.H35 2025 | DDC 617.7 H--dc23

TABLE OF CONTENTS

LIST OF ABBREVIATIONS

AAO	American Academy of Ophthalmology
AI	Artificial intelligence
AIOLIS	Assessment of Intraocular Lens Implant Symptoms
ALCOA+	Attributable, legible, contemporaneous, original, accurate, complete, consistent, enduring, and available
ASCRS	American Society of Cataract and Refractive Surgery
CITI	Collaborative Institutional Training Initiative
CRF	Case report form
CRN	Collaborative research network
CRO	Clinical research organization
CV	Curriculum vitae
EDC	Electronic data capture
ePRO	Electronic patient-reported outcomes
ETDRS	Early Treatment Diabetic Retinopathy Study
EMR	Electronic medical record
FDA	Food and Drug Administration
GCP	Good clinical practice

ICH	International Council for Harmonisation
ID	Identification
IEC	Independent ethics committee
IOL	Intraocular lens
IOP	Intraocular pressure
IRB	Institutional review board
IRIS	Intelligent Research in Sight
IT	Information technology
JCRS	*Journal of Cataract and Refractive Surgery*
LASIK	Laser-assisted in situ keratomileusis
logMAR	Logarithm of the minimum angle of resolution
MIG	Microinvasive glaucoma
MRSE	Manifest refraction spherical equivalent
MS	Microsoft
NIH	National Institutes of Health
POAG	Primary open-angle glaucoma
PRO	Patient-reported outcome
PROWL-SS	Patient-reported outcomes with LASIK symptoms and satisfaction
SAS	Statistical analysis system
SD	Standard deviation
SEO	Search engine optimization
UK	United Kingdom
VA	Visual acuity
WHO	World Health Organization

PREFACE

My name is Brad Hall. I am on a mission to simplify clinical research because I believe that more doctors doing good research leads to better medical care for everyone. I wrote this book to improve eye care and to help professionals bring those improvements to international attention.

I have been involved in research for more than 10 years and am the founder of Sengi, a clinical research organization (CRO), specializing in investigator-initiated trials in eye care. In 2024, Sengi supported 30-plus studies funded by leading ophthalmic companies such as Alcon, Johnson & Johnson, and Topcon. We're known for getting our clients published in medical journals and accepted to speak at conferences. In the past five years we have achieved success for our clients by leading their work through 35-plus publications in highly recognized journals, such as the *American Journal of Ophthalmology* and the *Journal of Cataract & Refractive Surgery*. With our expertise, our clients have peace of mind as we take care of all the paperwork so that they can focus on their patients.

This book is not a solicitation for Sengi, however. I believe that the best approach is for eye-care professionals to focus on optimizing clinical trials internally through their own management, but if needed, to turn to CROs with the needed expertise to assist with or entirely manage clinical trials for the professional. Either way, the payoffs are immense.

If you read all the way to the end, I promise that you'll understand how the LENS system, which is a four-step framework for success in clinical trials, can transform your eye-care practice.

INTRODUCTION

There has never been an easier time for eye-care professionals to conduct their own clinical trials. Just in the past year, Salus IRB, one of the more popular institutional review boards (IRBs) in the U.S., has finally moved completely to an online submission platform. So, gone are the days of applying for ethics approval with paper forms! Digital is replacing paper in other areas, too, as data can also be collected through electronic data capture (EDC) systems and web-based questionnaires. The digital age is empowering private practices to drive innovation in eye care—but not everyone is taking advantage.

The reality is that even with those advances, the extensive process to successfully complete research projects remains one of the most difficult times for eye-care professionals.

Ophthalmologists and optometrists not only have enormous amounts of patients to see but also must maintain all that's involved in running a busy practice. Hiring, training, and managing staff, plus collecting fees, paying bills, and purchasing supplies—the list of things to do never gets smaller, only larger…not to mention the effects of the competitive landscape that eye-care professionals face.

Despite those demands, eye-care professionals who embrace investigator-initiated trials will create a lasting impact. The clinical data they collect, analyze, and share on stage at conferences and publish in journals will improve medical care for everyone.

As a forward thinker, you understand this opportunity—and the obstacles. You probably already recognize the positive impact that clinical research can have on your patients and your practice. Still, you may have a few limiting beliefs that are getting in the way of completing your first or next research study. Do any of the following statements sound familiar?

"I may not know all that's involved, but I don't anticipate any problem in running a clinical trial. I believe that completing a clinical trial will be just like running my practice. I can do it with my own internal resources."

"The regulatory and publishing processes of clinical research are secondary tasks. I'll get around to them eventually."

"Research is only for large pharmaceutical companies or academics."

While some of those statements might be true for some professionals, the reality of the details needed to successfully complete a successful clinical trial usually turns out to be quite different. Take heart: There is a path forward. By following the "eye-dea" to impact framework presented here, you can remove the mask of limiting beliefs and see clearly that with the right mindset and tools, private practices can initiate their own studies, transform patient care, and create a lasting legacy in eye care.

I know that "eye-dea" is a playful pun—and I went back and forth about whether to include it. In the end, I found that it accurately characterizes what you and so many eye-care professionals have, which is vision, creativity, and the ability to lead innovation through research. This book offers you structure to take your ideas and make a lasting impact in eye care.

WHAT ARE KEY OPINION LEADERS DOING RIGHT?

Have you ever noticed how certain ophthalmologists and optometrists are key opinion leaders? They always seem to be invited on stage to give their perspectives on new technology that is not even available on the market yet. And when they speak, others listen.

Their research is published in top medical journals. Their practices have all the latest tools and treatments for enhanced patient care.

But how did they get to where they are?

It almost always starts with clinical research!

It doesn't necessarily start with large multicenter trials, however.

Many of the key opinion leaders in your field may have started by sponsoring their own research—for example, retrospective trials.

Retrospective clinical trials look backward at data that has already been collected.

In the day-to-day running of your practice, you record patient data all the time. You may just not realize it.

Your patient charts are a gold mine for new insights into care—all you have to do is go digging.

COMMON PROBLEMS PREVENTING SUCCESS IN CLINICAL RESEARCH

Being involved in clinical research for more than 10 years has given me unique insights into the common problems faced by eye-care professionals in their clinical trials.

The first is that eye-care professionals are overwhelmed and have difficulty understanding their data and clinical trial results. That obstacle can lead to wasted resources, poor clinical decisions, and reduced patient outcomes.

The second is that such professionals are overworked and can't stay on top of grant submissions, regulatory submissions, and publishing. Research is competitive, and delays can lead to loss of funding and missed opportunities for recognition.

The third is lack of differentiation in a competitive field—being unknown. The eye-care market is saturated, and if eye-care professionals can't stand out through research, they could see a decline in patient volume, decline in top talent, and possible business closure.

All three problems take a toll on their practices. In this book are all-too-common examples of lost opportunities for research success intertwined with real cases of industry recognition.

I will provide case studies throughout the book but note that identities have been changed. Here is a case study of prudent management of a clinical trial.

Amy is an ophthalmologist in private practice who collected a great amount of data on outcomes between two similar, but competing, intraocular lenses (IOLs). Amy's problem was that she was struggling with the complexity of the biostatistical analysis and the medical writing required to compare the results from these two IOLs for publication in a medical journal.

Recognizing the value in partnerships, Amy handed off the analysis and medical writing and focused instead on what mattered more—the patients. She enjoyed the reduction in stress from worrying about data and writing, and even better, the study was published in a top medical journal.

THE BIG PAYOFFS FOR OVERCOMING COMMON PROBLEMS

Amy tends to be an exception to those who attempt to muddle through but miss a successful outcome. There is good news, though. The three common problems mentioned above can be conquered and result in three big payoffs.

1. The first payoff is peace of mind that comes to eye-care professionals by having clear, actionable insights from their data that will lead to immediate improvements in decision-making for patient care.
2. Second, they will have smooth operations that provide relief from stress and time pressure, enabling their work to gain appreciation more quickly.
3. Third, they will gain recognition that will attract more patients, research opportunities, and collaborations.

The ultimate payoffs will be a strong reputation for successful clinical trials and meaningful contributions to eye care, high-quality publications, and an influential career that impacts both the medical community and patient outcomes on a broad scale.

WHAT THIS BOOK WILL TEACH YOU

By reading this book you will learn, in depth, the four-step framework for success in clinical trials that makes up the LENS system:

1. **L**aunch with focus. Efficiently develop a research idea, secure funding, and receive ethics approval so that you can get the project off the ground.
2. **E**nroll with confidence. Quickly recruit patients and have them complete all follow-up visits.
3. **N**otice the insights. Collect useful data and analyze it to answer the research questions.

4. **S**hare the results. Publish your research in a medical journal and get on stage to speak about your achievements at conferences.

Through the LENS system, eye-care professionals can get IRB approval in weeks—not months—which is a significant head start on enrollment to further accelerate timelines and thereby gain unique insights from their data as well as the advantage of improved visibility through a focus on conference presentations and peer-reviewed publications.

You'll also learn the entire process for conducting a successful clinical trial. This collaboration begins with proper design, completion of all the proper regulatory submissions, best practices for data collection, management, and analysis, and dissemination of the results of your study to your colleagues.

PART 1:

FOUNDATIONS FOR TURNING EYE-DEAS INTO IMPACT

CHAPTER 1: UNDERSTANDING THE LANDSCAPE OF INVESTIGATOR-INITIATED TRIALS

START WITH A SOLID FOUNDATION

We'll cover the LENS system, a signature framework to execute a successful investigator-initiated trial, in part 2. For now, let's build a solid foundation upon which to anchor the four steps. If you have conducted your own such studies already, you don't need to skip ahead. I am confident you'll find a few nuggets of actionable information in this chapter that you can use to improve upon your existing workflow.

This chapter will start with the very basics in answer to the question "What is an investigator-initiated trial?" The details will also outline, very basically, what is involved, and by the end of the chapter you will know whether conducting an investigator-initiated trial is right for your purposes.

WHAT IS AN INVESTIGATOR-INITIATED TRIAL?

In general, clinical trials are the means to bring to market new developments in drugs and devices. Clinical trials have four phases:

- Phase 1. Assess the safety, side effects, and correct dosage or application of a new drug or device
- Phase 2. Evaluate the efficacy of the drug or device while continuing to assess safety
- Phase 3. Compare to other standard treatments and confirm efficacy and monitor for side effects
- Phase 4. Collect real-world results of safety and efficacy of the drug or device **after** regulatory approval

Phases 1, 2, and 3 are sponsored by large pharmaceutical or device companies and cost hundreds of millions of dollars. To put things into perspective, the process costs almost US$1 billion to bring a new drug to market in the U.S., taking into account previous failures and capital costs![1]

In traditional or industry-sponsored clinical trials, the new drug or device needs to be tested in humans, but the sponsoring companies don't actually have patients of their own. Eye-care professionals are needed in order to successfully complete the trials that depend on sponsor support. Therefore, the company sponsoring the clinical trial hires a medical professional as an investigator, and the professional effectively works for the company during

1 Aylin Sertkaya et al., "Costs of Drug Development and Research and Development Intensity in the US, 2000–2018," *JAMA Network Open* 7, no. 6 (2024): e2415445, https://doi.org/10.1001/jamanetworkopen.2024.15445.

the trial. In that arrangement, the sponsors develop the research question, tell the professional what data to collect and when, and arrange to send clinical monitors to the site to observe the trial conduct and to review the collected data.

My focus in this book is centered on the studies conducted by eye-care professionals themselves with their patients. Unlike traditional clinical trials, investigator-initiated trials, as the name suggests, are launched and led by an investigator, not industry. There are different terms depending on the context (investigator-initiated studies, physician-led trials, and investigator-sponsored trials, investigator-sponsored research), but the model is generally the same, where the investigator acts as both the sponsor and the investigator.

Table 1. Key differences between traditional or industry-sponsored clinical trials and investigator-initiated trials

	Investigator-initiated trial	Industry-sponsored trial
Sponsor	Investigator	Company
Funding source	Unrestricted grant	Company
Study design control	High—investigator led	Low—company led
Publication rights	Investigator has full control	Company has full control
Regulatory responsibilities	Investigator	Company

Such trials fit under the umbrella of phase 4 studies, at which point the trials are usually—and almost always—done with already-approved products. Since the drug or device has already received regulatory approval, commencing a phase 4 study not only significantly decreases the cost but also has an added benefit in that the professional can remain independent of the sponsor. Professionals are then free to develop their own research question and to conduct and manage the clinical trial as they want, within standard ethical and regulatory frameworks (more about them later).

A lot of great advancements can be made by doing research with already-approved products. Here are a few examples:

- Gain real-world clinical data on the safety and efficacy of a drug or device
- Answer clinician-specific questions that were not addressed in earlier clinical trials
- Improve the workflow of a treatment or surgical technique
- Fill in knowledge gaps left by the phase 1, 2, and 3 studies

Let me give you a real-world example.

Ruby and Hazel are a dynamic duo in their optometry practice. Always striving for the best care, they wanted to objectively know if a newly available product would benefit their patients. These professionals decided to run their own experiment via their own clinical trial to find out. They had some research experience but had never conducted an investigator-initiated clinical trial. They partnered with an experienced CRO that walked them through developing a research question, applying for grant funding, conducting the study, and publishing the results in a medical journal. Since then, Ruby and Hazel have successfully completed three such trials (with more ongoing), published their influential research, and have become authoritative in their field.

An investigator-initiated trial is exactly as it sounds: You take on the role of the sponsor and the investigator. That responsibility may sound intimidating, but I can assure you that by reading this book you will have the knowledge and action steps to succeed and make an impact in your field of care.

WHAT IS INVOLVED WHEN CONDUCTING AN INVESTIGATOR-INITIATED TRIAL?

Now that you have a better idea of what an investigator-initiated trial is, let's discuss what is involved so that you know what to expect before jumping in. All of the topics discussed here appear later in this book in greater detail, but this section will provide a general overview of what is involved.

STEP 1: Develop a Research Question

The research question or hypothesis relates to the central objective of the study.

STEP 2: Draft the Study Protocol

The protocol is a formal document that summarizes your research question, how you are going to answer the question, what study population you need, what examinations and visits participants will need or attend, and how you will protect any participant's rights.

STEP 3: Create the Informed Consent Form

The consent form summarizes the study in plain language for the participants to read, understand, and agree to before any study-related procedures are performed.

STEP 4: Submit Documents for Approval

The protocol and informed consent need to be reviewed and approved by an official organization, such as an institutional review board (IRB) or independent ethics committee (IEC), before the trial can begin. The IRB or IEC will also review other key documents, which we will cover in depth in chapter 4.

STEP 5: Collect Data

With approval, you can start to recruit, screen, and enroll eligible participants. Study data can be collected on paper or electronic forms in what are called case report forms (CRFs). Strict requirements must be applied to ensure data accuracy and integrity (more on that in chapter 6).

STEP 6: Analyze Results

Once all the data has been collected, you can start a formal analysis. It will involve descriptive statistics (e.g., mean, median, standard deviation, range) and perhaps inferential statistics (e.g., comparisons between data and the infamous *p* value) if your study design calls for it.

STEP 7: Communicate Findings

Present the findings on stage at conferences or more formally in an article published in a peer-reviewed medical journal.

Now, let's talk about money. The "sponsor" in investigator-initiated trials is you—you are responsible for paying for the study. The funds don't have to come out of your own pocket (we'll review applying for grant funding in chapter 4), but you will need to cover all expenses. They might include these:

- The drug or device of your study, known as the investigational product
- The IRB or IEC review fees
- Patient compensation
- Staff and clinic resources
- Consultants or CROs

Any investigator-initiated study requires numerous roles that need to be filled to run a successful trial. One person can have multiple roles but beware of stretching people too thin or relying too heavily on internal resources if you don't already have sufficient expertise in house. Here is a list of a few key roles:

- Investigator. You! In charge of the conduct of the study
- Study coordinator. Main point of contact for participants in the study (the grease that keeps the trial moving forward)

- Regulatory coordinator. Prepares all the documents needed for regulatory approval and is the main point of contact with those entities
- Biostatistician. Best choice to determine the appropriate statistical tests and confirms that the target sample size will be adequate to answer the research question
- Medical writer. Prepares, submits, manages article submissions to medical journals, and produces slide presentations for conferences

Phew! Now, I trust that you have a better—albeit, brief—idea of what's involved. My intention is that laying out the overview plainly will take away a lot of the anxiety about running your own investigator-initiated trial. Keep reading because in part 2 we will review, in detail, each of the pieces above and how they fit into the LENS system.

IS RUNNING AN INVESTIGATOR-INITIATED TRIAL RIGHT FOR YOU?

Let me start by saying that plenty of eye-care professionals run successful practices without conducting clinical trials. However, if you are at all interested—and you must be because you are reading this book—then I assure you that you are more ready than you believe to conduct research!

If you are on the fence about doing research, know that the goal of this book is not to pressure you into running investigator-initiated trials but instead to offer a guide for success, should you so choose.

Everyone has different motivations for clinical research. Some want to validate their own innovative approaches to patient care, increase their reputation among colleagues and patients, or grow their practices. Almost all have curiosity and a desire to maximize outcomes for their patients.

The majority of investigator-initiated trials are typically conducted by eye-care professionals in private practice. Although university settings can work, too, those sites generally involve more red tape.

Regardless of the setting, however, there are five key elements required to successfully execute an investigator-initiated trial:

1. **Time** is probably the most critical aspect because it always seems to be in short supply. Sure, you can delegate a lot of tasks to staff or a third-party partner (such as a consultant or CRO), but you still need time to plan and oversee each trial.
2. **Money** is the second most crucial aspect. You can get started with a retrospective study for just a few thousand dollars if you take on most of the work in house (more on that in part 3).
3. **Team** takes third place because no one can do trials alone. At the very least, you should have a staff member act as the study coordinator, which is the main contact for all patients. Think of that role as the manager of the day-to-day operations of the study.
4. **Space**—that is, the need for adequate room for the study—might seem obvious, but it is worth mentioning.

You need a place to see patients and to store research-related items such as documents, investigational product (the drug or device). For eye-care professionals, for example, space means having a room with the right equipment and dimensions for visual acuity measurements.

5. **Experience** is an important factor to consider in taking on such studies, but if you are new to research, you can lean on partners such as your mentors, consultants, or CROs.

Beyond those considerations, another aspect to be aware of is any limiting belief(s) that hold you back from embarking on your clinical trial journey. Table 2 outlines a few common examples.

Table 2. Example of limiting beliefs versus reality

Belief	Reality
I am not affiliated with a university.	The vast majority of investigator research is done in private practice.
I don't have any money for research.	Retrospective clinical trials are a great way to start, costing just a few thousand dollars.
I am not a writer, statistician, or XYZ.	Research is a team sport. You can partner with experts.
I don't even know where to begin.	You have already started by picking up this book!
I am worried the project will fail.	Even studies that don't generate publishable data are an opportunity to learn and improve for next time.

Let's look at a hypothetical example.

Sofia began her investigator-initiated trial journey by using the data she had already collected during the course of routine practice.

That method is called a retrospective trial (more on it in part 3) and is, what I think, the best place to start. Her success in completing the retrospective trial led to grant funding for prospective trials and involvement in larger multicenter trials. Now, she completes multiple grant-funded studies per year, frequently publishes in medical journals, is on stage speaking to large audiences at conferences, and can offer the latest treatment options for her patients.

You have already started on the path to successful investigator-initiated studies by picking up this book. I trust that Sofia's example illustrates that you can start small and build up capabilities over time. Remember that research is a team sport—you don't have to take on everything yourself.

SELF-ASSESSMENT: ARE YOU READY FOR INVESTIGATOR-INITIATED TRIALS?

The following 10 questions are designed to help evaluate your current readiness to undertake a clinical trial and where you might need to improve. This self-assessment tool evaluates core capabilities that the LENS system will enhance. Answer honestly and know that there are no wrong answers. (If you are unsure, choose answer c).

1. What is your confidence level for your overall study design for your investigator-initiated trial?
    a. High. Our design meets all regulatory standards and is clearly defined.
    b. Moderate. We are not clear on a few points.
    c. Low. We're unsure if the design is optimal.

2. Will you be able to comply with the latest regulatory and ethical standards?
    a. Yes. We are up to date and compliant.
    b. Maybe. The standards are known to us, but we struggle to keep up to date and in compliance 100%.
    c. Not yet. We need help to get there.
3. When preparing clinical trial documentation (e.g., protocols, informed consent, CRFs), are you able to adhere to industry best practices?
    a. Yes. All of our forms are adherent.
    b. Mostly. We need help in certain areas.
    c. No. We need help with all of our documentation.
4. Is your informed consent form clear and easy to understand for participants?
    a. Yes. Participants can read and understand the risks and benefits of the study.
    b. Mostly. We struggle to simplify the language for participants.
    c. No. Our participants often find the forms confusing.
5. How effective are your recruitment efforts for clinical trials?
    a. Very. We have no trouble meeting enrollment goals.
    b. Somewhat. Our methods are working but could be improved.
    c. Not at all. We struggle to recruit participants for our trials.
6. Are you efficiently collecting data?
    a. Yes. We have a streamlined system that minimizes the time and effort required.
    b. Somewhat. Certain processes take up a lot of time.

   c. No. Data collection takes a lot longer than expected and often contains errors.

7. Speaking of errors—do you have a system in place to minimize, identify, and correct errors?
   a. Yes. Our data is clean and error-free.
   b. Mostly. Errors still appear in our datasets.
   c. No. We are plagued by data errors that lead to significant delays.
8. Does your statistical analysis plan align with your study design?
   a. Yes. The statistical methods will directly answer the research question.
   b. Mostly. We are unclear on the appropriate statistical tests for each comparison.
   c. No. We need a biostatistician to prepare it for us!
9. Are you able to confidently meet the submission requirements and guidelines for medical journals?
   a. Yes. We are familiar with the process.
   b. Somewhat. We have had both successes and failures in the past.
   c. No. We often face delays or outright rejections for not following guidelines.
10. How would you rate the quality of your visual aids (e.g., charts, graphs) when you speak at conferences or publish in medical journals?
   a. High. We often get positive feedback from peers.
   b. Moderate. We follow general guidelines but struggle to make our visual aids effective.
   c. Low. We are unaware of best practices.

Take a deep breath and look back through your answers. If you chose mostly *a*'s, congratulations! You are off to a great start. If you chose mostly *b*'s, you are on the right track. If you chose mostly *c*'s, don't worry! We all have to start somewhere, and we can only improve by knowing where we might be deficient. Whatever your score, keep up the good work, and keep reading for more information on how to run successful investigator-initiated trials and get the most out of them.

MAKE AN IMPACT

- Find one hour in your schedule next week to sit down and think about your burning clinical questions or gaps in knowledge that you could explore.
- Reach out to a colleague who has done research to chat about what is involved and ask any questions that you may have.
- Pick up the latest copy of your favorite medical journal and identify and review the details for one investigator-initiated study. Tip—usually, the source of funding is disclosed as a grant (or no funding is disclosed at all). Such information or lack thereof is how you can tell the studies are investigator initiated.

CHAPTER 2:
COMMON MISTAKES THAT LEAD TO TRIAL FAILURE

IGNORE INTIMIDATION—DON'T SIT ON THE SIDELINES

Clinical research is an exciting endeavor! Not only do you get to be at the cutting edge of knowledge, but you are also able to affect the lives of patients. In eye care, your contribution could reveal the benefits of implanting a new intraocular lens that restores spectacle independence for a cataract patient. Or maybe a new combination of improvements, such as a glaucoma eyedrop, that keeps patient compliance high and intraocular pressure low!

While clinical research can seem overwhelming, don't let fear stop you. Yes, the thought of being a part of a large multicenter clinical trial on a pivotal new drug or device might seem beyond your abilities, especially if you are unfamiliar with clinical research, but trust me. I will lead you through the process by providing sound advice to begin. Remember—you can start small!

I truly believe that the best way to start clinical research in eye care and to create a lasting impact is through investigator-initiated studies. With an investigator-initiated trial, you take on the role of both the investigator and sponsor, which means that not only do you get to be involved in clinical research, but you also get to have control. You get to decide what research question you want to answer and how to answer it! I personally think that this arrangement can be far more exciting and effective in eye care. Contrast it with traditional clinical trials, where the sponsor (such as a medical device or drug company) has control over the study, because they are paying for it!

As you delve into clinical research, realize that your journey can be fraught with mistakes if you are not prepared and careful. My goal in this section is to be your guide on what **not** to do. I have been involved in clinical research in eye care for 10-plus years and have discovered five key mistakes that lead to clinical trial failure. In this chapter, we will review each of them in detail. Armed with this information, you will be better positioned to avoid common mistakes and achieve clinical trial success.

MISTAKE 1: UNDERESTIMATING CLINICAL TRIAL COMPLEXITY

You are an expert in your field—there is no doubt about that. However, it is a mistake to think that because you run a private practice, you can easily manage a clinical trial. Clinical studies are complex, and each step has its own intricacies. Let me give an example of a colleague who underestimated the complexity of clinical trials.

Tim wanted to conduct a retrospective study. Not knowing what he did not know about the ethics of clinical research, he and his team went ahead and collected, analyzed, and reported data on participants from their patient population without first getting IRB or IEC approval for the study and approval to waive informed consent from patients. Not only were both requirements a huge lapse in ethical and related standards, but without both documents, the collected data became unusable for publication in a medical journal or even for presentation at a conference.

Had Tim appreciated the difficulties and complexities of clinical research, he would have understood that all research involving humans needs proper ethical oversight and formal approval. The biggest part is informed consent, even for a retrospective study.

Clinical trials are multifaceted. They include elements like protocol design, informed consent documents, IRB or IEC approval, patient recruitment, regulatory compliance, data analysis, and reporting. Oversimplification of clinical trials may leave you open to being hit by avoidable obstacles. Some of the complexities may not be that obvious, such as regulatory and ethical hurdles.

Yet, the obstacles can be overcome with knowledge. In fact, not acknowledging the intricate details behind clinical trials can lead to significant study delays. The amount of time to move forward in the study needs to be budgeted into the process. Be prepared to wait a few weeks to hear back from an IRB or IEC after you submit the necessary documents. Moreover, if you haven't prepared them correctly, you will have to start the process over again, causing significant and unnecessary delays. Too many delays here can lead to significant budget overruns.

Major missteps are not all that professionals need to consider because minor ethical issues can arise as well. Though minor issues may seem small, they can cause collected data to become unusable. For example, one concern is in not thinking enough about or understanding how the study protocol interplays with your clinic routine and patient population. Here's one example.

Manuel was conducting an investigator-initiated trial but failed to reconcile the study protocol with his patient population. The written inclusion and exclusion criteria left out a lot of potential participants, and he struggled to enroll participants. Ultimately, the grant funder canceled the study as the lack of recruitment caused significant delays.

Failing to fully grasp the complexities of clinical trials can hurt your reputation. What will your internal resources think about you when the IRB or IEC keeps rejecting your study? What will future sponsors or grant funders think about you if your site is reprimanded by the IRB or IEC for ethical lapses or if your site is shut down entirely? If you can't successfully complete a clinical trial, your career may stall, preventing the elevation of your medical practice.

In my experience, there are three traps that eye-care professionals fall into when they underestimate clinical trial complexity. The first is that they have only limited—or perhaps no—experience with clinical trials. Lack of experience can be overcome by learning from or by partnering with external experts—lacking experience while thinking that you can still run a trial on your own can be a problem.

The second common trap is overconfidence in existing systems. Clinical research is always changing, and what worked for you in the past might not work in the future. What was formerly fragmented storage of paper documents has led to electronic cloud storage solutions. CRFs, once prepared on paper, are now being replaced by electronic forms in EDC platforms such as REDCap. If you are unaware of the continual technological advancements, you will lose out on trial efficiency and data accuracy. Competitive sites that have streamlined their trials will ultimately gobble up all the sponsored trials and grant funding.

Here is a good example. Let's say you want to investigate patient-reported outcomes in your clinical trial. Let's assume that it's the only piece of data that you want to collect and analyze. A prior way of approaching the study might be to bring all the study participants into your practice, obtain their consent in person, and have them complete a paper questionnaire. Then, you'd take all the responses and manually enter them into a database. That method might be feasible for 40 participants, but how about for 10 times that amount? Using that method would cause a logistic nightmare and likely—or at least potentially—be disruptive to the day-to-day running of your practice. In this digital age, however, professionals can leverage technology and follow updated clinical trial practices by getting patient consent remotely and by providing an electronic questionnaire that automatically populates a database. Think of the time and resources that saves.

The last snare is a nonmedical definition of what's commonly known as tunnel vision, through which many eye-care professionals focus solely on attending to their patients and neglect to focus on the broader clinical research project. This situation can lead to inadequate allocation of enough time and resources for critical elements such as data management, regulatory compliance, and reporting.

Assuming you've avoided all the above issues, the next concern is to have the study details and conclusions written in scientific terms and in a format according to a publication's requirements. Here, the temptation is to delegate the writing of a clinical study report or scientific manuscript to junior eye-care professionals or residents. More often than not, delegation of that task does not work well or to your benefit. It is not because those individuals are not bright and capable but because such types of technical writing require specialized skills, which generally are developed only through higher education and by constant practice. Keep in mind the importance of seeking a professional writer to compose your study report or article for a medical journal.

Here's another client—we'll call him Henry—who underestimated the complexity of writing an article for submission to a medical journal. Henry let a resident prepare and submit it. Unfortunately, it lacked proper structure and citations, not to mention that it didn't provide a cohesive message, so it was rejected by the medical journal to which it was submitted. Not only were time and effort lost, but the opportunity to publish in that particular medical journal was lost because it and many journals do not allow resubmissions after rejection. What was worse was that all the effort lost to his poor decision also increased the chances that another practice would swoop in and publish a similar study, stealing all the glory.

Preventing the misfortune of underestimating the complexities of clinical trials is a choice you must make and one within your control if you wish to engage in clinical trials. The best advice is to partner with experts who have spent their careers in clinical research and will help you navigate any difficulties and obstacles that arise. With outside help, you will have peace of mind to focus on your patients.

MISTAKE 2: USING INADEQUATE DATA-MANAGEMENT TOOLS

Another eye-care professional, Rachel, while running an investigator-initiated trial, was trying to locate some missing data from the dataset that they had collected. As it turned out, study staff had been recording critical data on sticky notes—some of which were lost along with the data, never to be recovered. Rachel was disappointed at the loss of the data and was left with two options: Try and recruit more participants to offset the lost data, causing delays, or proceed with less data than anticipated for analysis, potentially leading to subpar results. Neither was a great choice.

Most people these days have heard the expression "Garbage in, garbage out." If you haven't heard of it, it's not literally about garbage. What it means is that if you try to do an analysis with bad data, you will get a bad result. Worse, you could get a completely wrong answer and make misinformed decisions in your medical practice. If you want good data, you need proper data-management practices.

I get it—running a busy medical practice leaves very little time to focus on data-management practices. But in terms of clinical trials, the reality is that you can make your situation much worse by ignoring data management, as the case above highlights. Clinical research success is dependent on accurate and efficient data. Without it, there is no point in running a clinical trial. After all the planning, execution, follow-up appointments, and resources spent, data is the deliverable.

Without good data, you're essentially running in place. Additionally, not focusing on data management can have huge financial impacts. Poor data management almost always—if not always—causes general delays in the clinical trial and can lead to cost overruns or even loss of funding from a third party. The biggest waste is in resources—think dollars, your time, your staff's time, clinic hours, and patients' time. With efficient data-management practices, you will spend less on resources to get better data from your clinical trial. Beyond the impact of costs, you'll free yourself and your staff to focus on other important tasks.

The nonfinancial impacts can be huge as well. Think about the impact to your reputation. You don't want to be known as a research site that produces junk data. What would your patients think if they knew you were so careless with their data and wasted their time? What would your colleagues think if they knew about your poor oversight and attention to detail? What would grant funders and sponsors think if they knew you wasted their time and money to get unusable data?

Poor data management in just one clinical trial can affect your ability to conduct future research, secure adequate funding, and get recognition. Those risks can be avoided, however, because inadequate data management generally has three sources attributable to those problems.

The first is a lack of proper systems and tools. The case example above where study staff were recording data on sticky notes is an alarming example of lack of attention to systems and tools. To conduct an efficient clinical trial, systems need to be in place to validate the data from examinations, record and store the data, and analyze the data. A breakdown in any one of these areas can harm your trial.

Here's another example: Alicia was running a clinical trial in eye care, where manifest refraction spherical equivalent (MRSE) was a key endpoint. After adding proper systems and tools, Alicia was able to learn that one study staff member was calculating MRSE by adding half the sphere to the cylinder, instead of adding half the cylinder to the sphere. If that error had not been caught, the data for this endpoint would have been nonsensical, and the success of the trial would have been in jeopardy.

Another problem and its source involve data overload. Without a sense of what key pieces of data are needed to answer the research question, the objective turns into a tendency to collect as much data as possible. Excessive data can make for a time-intensive and difficult process to extract the key pieces of information later. Unnecessary data also leads to the temptation to perform endless analyses by comparing every variable, thereby wasting resources and diluting key findings about the study endpoints.

In another study, Jill collected an enormous amount of data because of her primary interest in all conceivable comparisons. However, by understanding that the collection was a data overload, she was able to take a step back. She reassessed which key comparisons were relevant to the original research question and was able to cut down the original list of comparisons by two-thirds, gaining clarity as well as saving time and money.

The final source of the problem is lack of expertise. As an eye care professional, you are undoubtedly excellent in providing the best care for your patients. Data collection and treatment, however, are and should be distinct parts of your practice. Many professionals like yourself are unaware that data management has a lot of complexities and obscurities. Understanding data is often related to the saying "What you don't know, you don't know," which can seriously affect your clinical trial. One solution to that problem requires hours and hours of learning to look at data in the right way. The simpler and better approach is to bring in partners that specialize in data management. Sure, that partnering may seem like a large up-front cost, but trust me, the time, money, and clean data obtained will more than make up for the expense.

Consider, for instance, the inadequate data-analysis tools observed in the literature. Taking the responses on a Likert-type scale (very dissatisfied, dissatisfied, neutral, satisfied, very satisfied) and coding them as 1 through 5 for the analysis in order to be able to take an average (or mean) of all responses is typically meaningless to obtain sufficient understanding of how good or bad the responses are.[2] Let's say the average of all responses equals 2.5. What can that number tell you about whether the literature is worthwhile? After all, "dissatisfied-and-a-half" is nonsensical! If you bring in an expert biostatistician, they're likely to say a more appropriate approach would be to summarize the data using percentages (e.g., 90% of participants reported being very satisfied). Remember—garbage in, garbage out.

I'm sure that your goal is to gain an elevated medical practice through clinical research, but the outcome of your efforts requires excellent data management. All it takes is engaging the right systems, using the proper tools, and reducing data overload. Those factors are inherent to successful clinical trials and are best accomplished by partnering with experts.

MISTAKE 3: OVEREXTENDING RESOURCES

When conducting a clinical trial in private practice, it is very tempting to keep all study-related activities in house. Logically, that tendency seems to make sense to keep costs low and simultaneously to empower staff to develop new skills that can be used for future studies—in essence, to have complete control over the entire process. The reality, though, is that such thinking is flawed and has the very real risk of leading to poor outcomes.

2 Phillip A. Bishop and Robert L. Herron, "Use and Misuse of the Likert Item Responses and Other Ordinal Measures," *International Journal of Exercise Science* 8, no. 3, (2015): 297–302, https://doi.org/10.70252/LANZ1453.

Most eye-care professionals like you are busy running their medical practice. Your staff members also are busy with the day-to-day tasks. Can you really squeeze in the amount of your time necessary for a clinical trial? And what about your staff, who are also trying to complete trial-related tasks that require expertise and experience to navigate regulatory compliance, data management, and scientific publishing?

In previous sections we reviewed how knowledge gaps can create problems. Here, let's focus on problems more at the macro or organizational level. Stretching yourself and staff too thin can significantly slow down the clinical trial, putting the whole study at risk of being canceled. In addition, your team may suffer a reduction in overall productivity and morale from being overburdened. Overextending resources can also lead to a poor output from rushing and not paying enough attention to detail.

Consider the IRB or IEC process. A lengthy back-and-forth interaction with the IRB or IEC eats up time that could be spent on other tasks. Not paying enough attention to detail with the IRB or IEC process can result in costly mistakes such as increased review fees or corrective action.

Having a just-get-it-done or this-is-good-enough attitude may work in nonpractice areas, but it does not work for clinical trials, which require many different facets of specialized skill and expertise to perform well. Think overall project management, data analysis, regulatory compliance, and publishing in medical journals. Success will come from the recognition that clinical trials are not a side project but a highly regulated environment—one that requires a mindset of excellence, patience, and attention to detail.

Here's a typical scenario: Karen was struggling to get a study off the ground and get IRB approval to be able to recruit patients. The main issue was that the IRB was confused by the way the protocol was written and would not approve it without significant changes. Karen failed to create systems for quality control to find issues in the protocol or other documents **before** IRB submission. The lack of robust systems significantly delayed acquiring the first patient for the first visit. Worse, the delay involved a very real risk that the grant funder was going to cancel the project and request the money back! Karen should have created internal processes for IRB submissions and approvals or even brought in external partners. In this case, overextending internal resources was more costly than hiring outside help!

An often-overlooked problem resulting from overextending resources is the long-term impact. First of all, time spent on clinical trial activities that could be outsourced becomes time not spent on developing the business and building relationships with sponsors, patients, and colleagues. The long-term effect becomes the inability to attract and execute much larger clinical trials. By partnering with companies that specialize in clinical trial activities, you will have dedicated time to focus on your business and your patients.

Don't fall for the idea that outsourcing the details of a clinical trial is a mistake or is a sign of **weakness**. You wouldn't consider that outsourcing tax preparation to an accountant showed weakness. Likewise, you wouldn't believe that outsourcing legal contracts to a lawyer is a mistake. Both such decisions are a sign of a strong leader, one who knows how to delegate tasks outside their own expertise. Letting the experts focus on what they do best allows you to focus on what you do best: patient care.

The same approach to partner with experts who have specialized knowledge and experience with all the associated work ensures that you will have much greater success with your study.

MISTAKE 4: VIEWING CLINICAL TRIALS AS LOW-PRIORITY SIDE PROJECTS

Let's look at the experience of Grace, who is a brilliant cataract and refractive surgeon. She made a good decision to conduct an investigator-initiated trial, but in her busy practice, she never seemed to dedicate enough time to the study's requirements. She treated it as merely a side project while she focused on other aspects of her practice—an all-too-common mindset.

During the course of the project, she experienced delays in getting IRB approval and subsequent delays in recruiting patients and completing all follow-up appointments. Moreover, on top of those issues, significant errors occurred in data collection and management. The result was that the study was unpublishable in a medical journal. Not only had too much time passed because of the approval delays and the other data issues, but she learned that other surgeons already had published their findings on the topic. In the end, the study she sought to complete turned into wasted resources with no real benefit to her practice. Grace was left financially and emotionally drained.

Grace's mistake is not an isolated one. Many eye-care professionals who start clinical trials often treat them like side projects. Certainly, patient care is a top priority, but the mistake is in thinking that clinical trials detract from patient care.

Such thinking is likely compounded by a lack of internal resources on top of the complexity of clinical trials. Unfortunately, treating clinical trials like a side project and not prioritizing them, as Grace's example illustrates, leads to wasted internal and external resources.

In addition, the poor outcome reflects badly on the reputation of the investigator to execute a successful trial and will affect future funding and collaboration opportunities. The effect in the longer term impairs access to cutting-edge treatments, such as those still in clinical trials or otherwise only available to a select few clinics. Furthermore, those consequences directly affect the investigator's continued excellence in patient care. All of those reasons are why I argue that successful clinical trials directly **improve** patient care and outcomes.

The point is to learn from and apply the lessons in the example above. You can gain huge benefits from prioritizing clinical trials in your medical practice. For one, you will have a competitive advantage over other eye-care practices. As a patient myself, I have an enormous choice of where to go for my eye-care needs. I want to go where I will receive the best care. To me, that choice focuses only on particular practices that regularly conduct research and have access to and are familiar with the latest innovations. Both of those qualities come from conducting clinical trials. In addition, successfully executing clinical trials and sharing the results in a medical journal or on stage at a conference builds visibility and credibility with peers, sponsors, and potential partners, not to mention how this develops your status as a highly regarded practice. You could also become a key opinion leader and a trusted expert in your field.

To access those benefits requires a mindset shift from thinking that clinical trials are a side project to understanding their strategic importance. Your thinking must instead focus on the long-term rewards of access to the latest innovations, improved patient care, and the boost to your professional reputation. It might not be easy to shift your mindset, but keep in mind that clinical trials are an investment in your future, the future of your medical practice, and future patient care. As you change your own mindset, you will need to foster a research-minded culture with your team, which will likewise benefit their future.

A number of steps can be taken immediately to start prioritizing clinical trials in your medical practice. The one that will have the largest impact is to build a dedicated research team whose primary focus is research. I know that in many practices, staff are already struggling with overwork (i.e., too many tasks and not enough time to complete them). But establishing a dedicated research team doesn't have to mean the group consists of all internal staff. The option exists to employ consultants, CROs, and other companies with which you can partner to reduce or eliminate the strain on internal resources. That being said, having a dedicated study coordinator in house is highly recommended. A study coordinator will develop a deep understanding of any study protocol and become a source of great help with recruitment, scheduling, managing paperwork, and the day-to-day operations of clinical trials.

Here's an example of a professional who understood how to leverage his resources. Xavier runs clinical trials at his medical practice like a well-oiled machine. He has a dedicated study coordinator in house who is solely responsible for all the ongoing clinical trials. Through the study coordinator's leadership, internal staff have become knowledgeable and now have experience with the IRB process. They routinely receive the green light for approvals in relatively short order. Then, once all the patient data is collected, those individuals hand it off to a CRO, which does all the analysis, reporting, conference preparation, and writing of the articles for publication in a medical journal. In fact, Xavier's talks about the findings of his research at conferences routinely win Best Paper, and his studies are published in the top medical journals of his field.

As a result of the many successful clinical trials run by Xavier and his dedicated team, sponsors and colleagues are constantly in contact with his practice about new trials and collaboration opportunities. With the many ongoing trials, Xavier has access to the latest innovations in eye care and can offer the best available care to his patients. Word gets around too. His practice is known for offering the best care in the area, and Xavier enjoys the peace of mind that financial stability brings.

Consider the examples of Grace and Xavier. Does one example reflect better on where you are now or where you want to be moving forward? Grace's failure or Xavier's success can be yours. If you want success in clinical trials, then start by treating them as an investment. You can accomplish this mindset shift today.

I also encourage you to commit this year to doing one new clinical trial and building your research team. Find a dedicated study coordinator and reach out to a few CROs and consultants to partner with. Through well-executed clinical trials you will build visibility, credibility, and recognition, have access to the latest innovations, and be able to provide the best available care to your patients. Remember that by prioritizing clinical research, you **are** prioritizing patient care.

MISTAKE 5: NOT PRIORITIZING PATIENT RECRUITMENT AND RETENTION

Another professional, Riley, was conducting an investigator-initiated trial in eye care. His practice was achieving great results for its patients, but Riley assumed that he would be successful without making patient recruitment a priority. The study was supposed to last less than one year, including follow-up, but when that deadline approached, only 10% of the total targeted participants had been recruited! Ultimately, support was pulled by the grant funder, and the project was canceled. An enormous amount of resources and effort was wasted in securing funding and getting the trial off the ground. Beyond those failures, the burden on staff to enroll patients in the study was all for naught, as 10% of the targeted recruitment did not equate into enough data to publish in a medical journal or to present at a conference, leading to significant burnout.

David, also an experienced professional, was likewise conducting an investigator-initiated trial in eye care. Unlike Riley, David's team was able to recruit all the necessary patients. However, many of the patients failed to return for their follow-up appointments after surgery. As a result, the sample size dropped below clinical relevance. The surgical outcomes were good, but with a smaller than targeted final sample size, the study lost a lot of impact. The grant funder in this situation also clawed back some of the given money due to the failure to achieve the target sample size. Again, time-consuming effort and resources were lost—even more so than those in Riley's study because David had recruited more patients overall but didn't prioritize the follow-up visits.

Both Riley's and David's stories illustrate a key mistake that many eye-care professionals make. Prioritizing patient recruitment and retention are not side tasks but are essential for clinical trial success. It is easy to get tunnel vision and focus on other tasks such as regulatory compliance, but without enough patients in recruitment and retention, the needed data isn't captured. It is also too easy to think that members of your existing patient population will sign up for the trial without too much effort by the practice or that they will stick around and attend all follow-up visits. On the contrary, enough time must be dedicated and budgeted to recruitment and retention of participants to enable the collection of good data and, ultimately, clinical trial success.

When eye-care professionals fail to prioritize patient recruitment and retention in a trial, the cost can be truly enormous. The greatest cost in all areas, as Riley's story demonstrates, stems from delayed timelines. Not only do delays increase costs as the trial pushes out the deadline, but the effect puts the entire study at risk if timelines are stretched too far and funding is pulled. In addition, as David's story illustrates, the quality and quantity of data are affected by dropouts. High attrition rates reduce the sample size for the study endpoints and reduce both statistical significance (probability that results are due to chance) and clinical significance (practicality of the results). Below a certain threshold, the data collected is unable to answer the overall study question, and the trial becomes a failure unless more patients are recruited to increase the sample size. The dilemma leaves eye-care professionals with a difficult decision: Cancel the trial and lose all the time and resources already put into it, or pour in more time and resources with the hope that enough new patients will complete all follow-up visits. Keep in mind that the latter choice is always time sensitive.

At a study's core, two main problems affect patient recruitment and retention for eye-care professionals.

The first is a focus on a passive approach to recruitment. Many eye-care professionals rely on their existing patient populations to be participants in an investigator-initiated trial. Recruitment is typically done when patients come into the practice for a routine checkup. With that passive approach, recruitment is often slower than anticipated, dragging out timelines and increasing costs. By contrast, a more active and, I would argue, more successful approach would be to also reach out to your patient population directly over the phone or to partner with other practices to have them refer eligible patients to you. (I will cover recruitment beyond your own practice in chapter 5.)

The second problem is weak patient engagement. Once patients are recruited, often there is very little ongoing communication with participants by the study staff, which can cause patients to feel disengaged and leave the study prematurely.

Both problems can be overcome by creating a patient-centered approach to clinical trials. First, you must put yourself into your patients' shoes and understand their motivation for wanting to participate and to complete all visits for your clinical trial. If you were a patient, what benefits would incentivize you to participate and comply? In general, patients need clearly articulated benefits and a sense of impact beyond just the research. Think about how answering the study question will affect future patient care, then formulate a statement about the potential outcome that will be meaningful to them—that context has enormous impact on their willingness to sign up.

Regarding benefits to patients, an obvious first step is monetary compensation for participation, which would include a dollar value for their time (including travel time), parking, and any overnight stays. I typically see compensation between $150 to $300 per participant for investigator-initiated trials in eye care.

Prioritizing patient recruitment and retention clearly affords huge benefits that await you and your practice.

The first benefit is the financial and operational boost. Faster recruitment speeds up timelines, which not only reduces costs but also has the added advantage of your team being first to publish. Consider the impact attached to a new treatment on the market.

Eye-care professionals who publish their results before others often get articles in top medical journals just by being first to report!

Second, patients will experience better outcomes. Have you ever noticed in your medical practice how patients who take an active role in their own care tend to have better outcomes compared to patients who don't?[3] Well, the same conclusion is true for clinical trials. Research has shown that the patients who remain engaged throughout a clinical trial will generally have better overall health outcomes.[4] Not only do such outcomes have a huge impact in the lives of your patients, but they also directly affect you because the reported results from your study will be better, which can boost the credibility of the research and your medical practice overall.

Last, your reputation will never be the same—in a good way. If you have ever wanted to be a part of a clinical trial for an **unapproved** device or drug, then you need to have a positive reputation in your field. If you are known to be a practice that excels at patient recruitment and retention, your practice will become more competitive for future traditional clinical trials. In addition, you will attract more opportunities for collaboration and funding for continued investigator-initiated trials.

3 Jessica Greene and Judith H. Hibbard, "Why Does Patient Activation Matter? An Examination of the Relationships Between Patient Activation and Health-Related Outcomes," *Journal of General Internal Medicine* 27, no. 5 (2012): 520–26, https://doi.org/10.1007/s11606-011-1931-2.

4 Fabio Dennstädt et al., "Patient Autonomy and Shared Decision-Making in the Context of Clinical Trial Participation," *European Journal of Clinical Investigation* 54, no. 11 (2024): e14291, https://doi.org/10.1111/eci.14291.

I encourage you to make patient recruitment and retention a core component of your clinical trial strategy. Not only will you improve the success of your clinical trial, but you will also enhance your connection to and your care of patients, advance your medical practice, and even influence the future of eye care.

MAKE AN IMPACT

- Review your internal resources and consider partnering with experts who have specialized knowledge and experience in clinical trials.
- Commit this year to building your research team and then doing one new clinical trial.
- Make patient recruitment and retention a core component of your clinical trial strategy to enhance patient care.

CHAPTER 3:
THE PAYOFFS OF RESEARCH DONE RIGHT

DECISION TURNING POINT

Three simple questions will help you decide whether you should pursue an investigator-initiated trial in eye care.

1. Are you interested in gaining recognition from colleagues?
2. Would you like to bring in more money for your clinic?
3. Do you want to increase the level of care that you can offer your patients?

All of those benefits and more—like becoming a key opinion leader or having access to the latest technological breakthroughs in your clinic—are available when you execute a successful clinical trial!

This chapter will cover five big payoffs. Read on to see how investigator-initiated trials can help you grow your practice, expand your income streams, increase your professional reputation, improve patient care, and become a preferred site for future trials.

PAYOFF 1: STAND OUT IN A CROWDED MARKET

Imagine you are a patient seeking eye care. You live in a moderately sized city, where ample choices are available to get the best care. But how do you choose? One strategy is to pick the closest private practice to where you are located, but because you live in the city, a lot of options still exist within a short drive. Your next priority, after location, is the level of care you will receive. Doing a little online research of the five nearest practices and talking with friends and family reveal that only one practice seems to offer cutting-edge treatment options and diagnostic equipment. In addition, the lead professional has a reputation for being involved in clinical trials, with access to additional advanced treatment options. This eye-care practice stands out in the crowded field in your city, so you book your first appointment with them as soon as possible.

That scenario shows that, in order to stand out in a competitive and saturated market, you should make clinical research a strategic asset because it will be a key differentiator. It will set your practice apart, help to accelerate growth, and enhance the traditional methods of attracting new patients through local advertising and word of mouth. Relying solely on advertising and word of mouth limits your visibility as you may appear to be just like all the other practices in your market. Worse, you could be seen as outdated if you are not including the latest treatments in your advertising. The true risk of not being able to set your practice apart from competition is an ultimate decline in patient volume and revenue.

In contrast, participating in clinical trials allows access to and encourages the use of cutting-edge innovations in eye care. Being up to date in your practice area is a vital asset that will set you apart from the competition. Patients want the best care, and they often associate new with better. If their friends and family are talking about the latest intraocular lens or vision-correction procedure, they will want the same treatment too. Regular participation in research also will give you a reputation as a leader in your field. If you are regularly completing clinical trials and communicating the results through publishing, speaking at conferences, and notifying your patients and the general public about your research, your status will help you to stand out in your community and in your industry. You will be positioned as a cutting-edge provider.

To advance your status as a patient-preferred provider, clinical research encourages the use of a patient-centered experience—that is, putting yourself into your patients' shoes to understand their motivations and give them the experience that they want. For example, regular check-ins with study participants are key to a successful clinical trial as the message encourages participants to complete all follow-up visits. Likewise, regular check-ins with your patient population can create an engaging experience that boosts patient loyalty, retention, and recommendations to others. Not only is regular communication a great choice to keep existing patients, but a patient-centered experience in a clinical trial also creates positive word of mouth at no cost to you. Further, by being regularly involved in clinical research, your practice's credibility with patients will be reinforced.

To patients, most practices can seem the same—or worse, they all may even blur together. Clinical research brings your clinic into sharp focus, amplifying your visibility, credibility, and value to patients.

PAYOFF 2: DIVERSIFY REVENUE STREAMS

In 2024, several U.S. Medicare administrative contractors imposed limitations for coverage of combined cataract and microinvasive glaucoma surgeries.[5] Not only is their decision misguided in terms of the recent research that shows the effectiveness of combining procedures, but it also has the consequence of limiting what medical procedures are covered. The restriction directly affects already strained revenues for ophthalmology practices as fewer patients will consider—or be able to afford—combined procedures if patients have to pay more out of pocket.

Now more than ever, eye-care practices need multiple income streams to balance out the chaotic and uninformed decisions made by bureaucrats. Income from many different sources reduces risk, stabilizes revenue, and can also provide growth opportunities.

Clinical trials are often overlooked but provide an invaluable source of diversification. An enormous amount of money is spent every year by companies trying to get new drugs or

5 "Micro-Invasive Glaucoma Surgery (MIGS)," Centers for Medicare and Medicaid Services, last updated March 27, 2025, https://www.cms.gov/medicare-coverage-database/view/lcd.aspx?lcdid=37578.

devices approved by health authorities such as the Food and Drug Administration (FDA). A lot of that money is spent on clinical research, with a large portion of the funds going to medical practices and investigators to conduct the trials. In addition, many medical device and drug companies will fund research projects on already-approved devices because it gives them evidence to back up any marketing claims—especially if it shows that their product is better than their competitor's. These are typically called investigator-initiated trial (or study) grants. State or provincial and federal grants also are available to medical practices to conduct research. All in all, money is available for eye-care practices that conduct clinical research. Despite these opportunities, evidence suggests that about one in 10 physicians are involved in clinical research.[6]

To get access to those research dollars, you need to position yourself as a site that gets reliable data in a reasonable time frame, which is most frequently done through successfully completing clinical trials and publishing the results. Now, you might be thinking, "Hold on—I need clinical research experience before I can get access to clinical trials? How am I supposed to do that?" The answer is that you can sponsor your own clinical trials, in which you are both the sponsor and investigator.

Another trickle-down effect of completing clinical trials to diversify your income is that you will develop a reputation for innovation. Being involved in cutting-edge trials gives your practice credibility and will attract patients who are interested in the latest

6 Jatin M. Vyas and Katrina A. Armstrong, "Physician-Scientist to Research-Engaged Physician—What Is in a Name?," *JAMA Network Open* 7, no. 9 (2024): e2433123, https://doi.org/10.1001/jamanetworkopen.2024.33123.

and best treatments. In general, 88% of patients would value being told about clinical research opportunities, but only 22% are.[7] There is opportunity for your practice to fill this gap. In addition, by having access to the latest treatments you can "niche down" (specialize) in helping patients who need specific care. Both avenues help you to stand out in a crowded and saturated market.

Through an investigator-initiated trial, Daniel discovered a nomogram (which is a formula that takes patient measurements and outputs a treatment plan) to help cataract and refractive surgeons select the most appropriate lens to implant in an eye. As a result of his discovery, his practice was able to diversify its income stream by licensing the data insights to colleagues, industry partners, or academic institutions.

Likewise, Elena also found diversified income through clinical trials. Through investigator-initiated research, she and her team developed an innovative software application to streamline data collection. They also have the option to license the data insights to colleagues, industry partners, or academic institutions.

We live in uncertain financial times, one where policies can change overnight. If you want to de-risk your practice, stabilize revenues, and find other avenues for growth, then focus on developing clinical research as a strategic asset.

7 Annick Anderson, Deborah Borfitz, and Kenneth Getz, "Global Public Attitudes About Clinical Research and Patient Experiences with Clinical Trials," *JAMA Network Open* 1, no. 6 (2018): e182969, https://doi.org/10.1001/jamanetworkopen.2018.2969.

PAYOFF 3: ACHIEVE GREATER PROFESSIONAL CREDIBILITY AND INFLUENCE

Being "invisible" in your field will not elevate your medical practice. In today's competitive world, if you are not standing out through professional recognition, then you are being left behind. An eye-care professional who remains invisible will see their colleagues surpass them by becoming key opinion leaders and securing more funding opportunities for their practice.

Charles had ambitions to be involved in sponsored clinical trials from top ophthalmology companies this year. He wanted to be able to access the latest devices and drugs for his patients. The problem? He and his practice were unknown and unproven. He had few to no published articles, and no one was seeing him give talks at conferences, despite the great results his practice was achieving for its patients. Soon after he started to publish the results in medical journals, however, his practice was being approached by colleagues and sponsors to partner on large multicenter clinical trials!

Eye-care professionals who keep a low profile, thinking that their great results will speak for them, are missing out on so many wonderful opportunities. By remaining unknown, they miss speaking engagements, leadership roles in their specialty, and invitations to be involved in clinical trials. Professionals who fall into that category stifle their own growth and the growth of their medical practice.

Professional recognition matters for three big reasons. First, it establishes a reputation for excellence. Colleagues, grant funders, staff, and patients all have evidence that you are committed to clinical trials in an effort to deliver the best patient care possible. As a patient myself, I would prefer to see an eye-care professional who is active in research because then I know that they are informed about the latest treatments, what works, and what doesn't work. I trust that I will get the best patient care possible.

Speaking of trust, professional recognition builds trust not only with patients but also with collaborators and sponsors. Recognition builds authority and credibility. For both collaborators and sponsors, having a track record of successful clinical trials signals that you can manage the complexity of clinical trials and generate meaningful data. Clinical trials require significant time, money, and resources, so having credibility through professional recognition makes it easier for others to decide to collaborate with you.

Last, professional recognition will open so many new doors for you. Once you become recognized in your field, you will gain access to larger clinical trials through bigger grants and sponsored trials. You will have device and drug companies coming to you and your practice to use and evaluate their cutting-edge products. You also will attract and retain a great team of staff around you.

Here is some more great news to help you in your decision to begin investigator-initiated trials. As you start to gain professional recognition, you'll see a ripple effect that will affect you and your medical practice. The first effect is career growth. Think in terms of key opinion leaders on stage at conferences. When they speak, the industry listens. You could be one. Professional recognition will lead to more collaboration opportunities, bigger clinical trials, and invitations to industry advisory boards. The remaining ripple effects are long-term benefits. They include increased career security, demand from industry and colleagues for your expertise, and a large and long-lasting impact in your field overall.

Through my 10-plus years in clinical research, I have noticed three big mistakes that eye-care professionals make that hold them back from building professional recognition.

The first is being too passive. You must not wait around to broadcast your success in research or expect your colleagues, large clinical trial sponsors, and patients to know that the work you do is top-notch. Sure, each individual patient may know, but prospective patients don't. If you want to attract more opportunities, you have to become active and start telling people about the results you are achieving.

Staying silent about your work is a trap that many professionals step in. See if you identify with Aria, who was silently sitting on a mountain of value and didn't recognize its importance in promoting her practice. Over time, she had collected an enormous amount of data through her private practice but hadn't published any of the results. She dreamed of working with key sponsors on important clinical trials, but her unpublished work remained invisible. Aria eventually made a concentrated effort to prioritize speaking at conferences and began to publish her research. The recognition she gained by focusing on both channels has had a huge impact on her career. Now, Aria and her team are working on multiple key clinical trials simultaneously for huge sponsors!

Another big mistake in building professional recognition is focusing only on publishing in medical journals. While this activity is key to increasing recognition, focusing all your energy there is a problem. For one, not all colleagues, industry players, and grant funders—and especially patients—read academic publications in medical journals. It is equally important for you to get on stage speaking at conferences so that at least your peers and potential partners can put a face to a name, as Aria's example illustrates. Such engagements really accelerate credibility and build trust. Think of the key opinion leaders in your field. Don't they always seem to be on stage talking about their research? (Conferences are also a great opportunity to network and find your next big project!)

The ultimate big mistake relates directly to the first two. It is giving into fear. Many eye-care professionals avoid publishing their research in medical journals or are unwilling to speak at a conference because they are afraid of what might happen. Their motive is threefold: to avoid being criticized, making mistakes, or receiving judgment. One particularly good piece of advice I received early on in my career was that making a mistake or being criticized, though uncomfortable, is really just an opportunity to improve. When peer reviewers of a manuscript write comments that poke holes in it, their input is not done maliciously. It is because they want your article to be the best paper possible. All such comments are an opportunity to learn and improve so that you don't make the same mistakes again.

Professional recognition is well within your reach. If you decide to grasp it and become more visible, you will attract more opportunities and partnerships. Keep in mind that seeking recognition for vanity's sake is not strategy for long-term success. The goal of gaining professional recognition is to grow yourself and your practice so that you can continuously offer the best care for your patients.

PAYOFF 4: EXPAND TREATMENT OPTIONS FOR PATIENTS

Investigator-initiated studies can help to grow your practice and provide additional treatment options for patients. First of all, if you secure support from a medical device or drug company, often you can get their treatment for no cost as part of the grant funding. That allowance also means that there would be potentially no cost to patients for the treatment either. The offer benefits them as well by allowing new treatments to be available for patients who might not otherwise be able to afford them. The funding may also partially or fully pay for extra equipment (such as basic or advanced diagnostic devices) for your practice.

For example, Joey was conducting an investigator-initiated trial of a new treatment, which was funded by a grant from an industry partner. As part of the grant, Joey was able to have on loan a diagnostic device that his practice could use to expand its patient care. Moreover, the loaner allowed him to test the device to see if it was able to improve care for his patients before the need to spend tens of thousands of dollars to purchase it. (It did!) That trade-off created a win-win situation.

Patient care is also expanded by the advance of research through clinical trials. Many investigator-initiated trials compare different treatments to determine which works best in particular patient populations. The answers to such questions not only improve the patient care of your own practice but also the care within those of your colleagues. For example, the ability to compare power-calculation formulas of intraocular lenses for accuracy in long- and short-axial length eyes, compare glaucoma therapies, or compare diagnostic equipment or surgical microscopes all serve to uncover better outcomes for patients.

Investigator-initiated trials are a great path to expand the treatment options that you offer to your patients. Prioritizing research ensures that you can continuously offer the best care for your patients.

PAYOFF 5: BECOME A PREFERRED SITE FOR FUTURE TRIALS

Investigator-initiated trials are a great way to establish yourself as a go-to site for future clinical trials. Not only will collaborators be more likely to provide grant funding for future investigator-initiated trials, but you also open up the possibility of being selected for large multicenter trials of not-yet-approved treatment options. If you want to reap those benefits, then you need to show a history of excellent performance and successful clinical trials. Conducting investigator-initiated studies is a great way to hone your clinical trial operations and start building a track record of success. This is a first step toward being invited to participate in multicenter trials for yet-to-be-approved medical devices and drugs.

Sponsors of FDA trials have a lot invested in the development of a device or drug, and often the pivotal multicenter trials have budgets in the millions of dollars. Therefore, these sponsors are understandably hesitant to work with sites and investigators with no clinical experience. They know from experience there is just too much that can go wrong and too much at stake.

By conducting successful investigator-initiated trials, you showcase that you and your site can recruit patients and meet enrollment targets and, better yet, that you can gather good data and maintain its integrity as well as showcase your history of meeting deadlines. Through successful studies, you perfect your clinic workflow (such as patient screening or document storage), acquire necessary equipment you might not otherwise have (such as a light meter or specialized diagnostic equipment), and get your staff much needed experience.

Everybody has to start somewhere. Eye-care professionals—like Sofia from chapter 1—who have followed the four steps of the LENS system now have sponsors banging down the front door of such practices to work with them on more investigator-initiated trials and to participate in pivotal clinical trials of yet-to-be-approved devices and drugs.

Since eye care is all about eyesight, imagine being in a pitch-black room. Each successful investigator-initiated trial you complete raises the light level a little. Eventually, grant funders, sponsors, and collaborators will begin to clearly see your ability to successfully conduct a trial—establishing you as a go-to site for future clinical trials.

MAKE AN IMPACT

- Set aside some time and review the current services that you offer. Identify what research opportunities would be the best fit with what you already specialize in.
- Create a research curriculum vitae (CV), which is like a regular CV, but it also outlines all your past research activities in a stand-alone section. Keep it updated with successful trials and post it on your practice's web page or other sites where you are a member, if allowed.
- Imagine you are giving a talk to your colleagues at a conference. Write down the title of your presentation, and as time allows, fill in the details you would include in it in anticipation of being invited to present at a conference.

PART 2:

MASTERING THE METHODS BEHIND IMPACTFUL TRIALS

CHAPTER 4:
LAUNCH WITH FOCUS

START TO FINISH

Moving from insight to impact can have an enormous positive influence on you, your staff, and your patients. I have helped many clients with no prior research experience start, execute, and communicate their first clinical trial. Through this work, I have developed the LENS system, a signature framework to take you from research idea to professional recognition. There are just four pieces of the puzzle.

The first is Launch with Focus—which is your ability to efficiently develop a research idea, secure funding, and receive IRB or IEC approval so that you can get the project off the ground. If you can't go from insight to recruiting patients quickly, your ideas will become papers that your colleagues write and speak about at conferences, while you are left thinking, "I thought about that first!" But implementation is more important than ideas. Anyone can have a great idea, but the greatest impact will be seen by those eye-care professionals who can take an idea, create a project, and get it off the ground.

As a companion to this book, I have created resources and templates for the documents discussed in this chapter, available at https://sengiclinical.com/eyedeatoimpact.

When you have an efficient start-up process, you will have better ideas, secure more grant funding, and be quicker to start recruiting patients.

HOW TO DESIGN A SUCCESSFUL INVESTIGATOR-INITIATED TRIAL

At this stage you will formulate your research question, choose the type of study, and determine the methodology you will use to answer the research question.

Your Research Question

The first step to design a clinical trial is to figure out what research question you want to answer. A good place to start is to investigate what is already published to see if you can identify a gap in the literature.

You can start by reading the top-three medical journals in your field to get your creative juices flowing.

Here are a few additional prompts to consider:

1. A new drug or device has become available, and you want to report on the clinical outcomes from your practice.

2. You have a unique patient population (e.g., long-term outcomes with a drug or device, age, race, environmental conditions).
3. You already have a large amount of data on a particular outcome.

Next, head on over to PubMed (https://pubmed.ncbi.nlm.nih.gov/) and double-check that your study idea has not already been published. If it has, keep iterating with reading journal articles and coming up with ideas. Eventually, you will find your big idea.

Choose Your Type of Study

There are five big items to consider when designing your study type:

1. Study arms. Will your study consist of a single arm (one group) or multiple arms (multiple groups)? Will one of the groups be a control group?
2. Masking. If there are multiple arms, will the investigators or patients or both be masked?
3. Randomization. Again, if there are multiple arms, will patients be randomly assigned to a treatment group?
4. Study sites or investigators. Will you be pulling data only from your patient population, or will you bring in collaborators from other practices to be subinvestigators?
5. Time period. Will your study collect data going forward (prospectively), backward (retrospectively), or a combination (referred to as ambispectively)?

Endpoints

Study endpoints are the specific outcomes that you will measure to answer the research question. For example, if the purpose of your study is to measure visual outcomes after implantation of a new presbyopia-correcting intraocular lens, then your endpoints might be one of these:

- Uncorrected distance visual acuity (logMAR) three months postoperatively
- Corrected distance visual acuity (logMAR) three months postoperatively
- Uncorrected intermediate visual acuity (logMAR) three months postoperatively
- Uncorrected near visual acuity (logMAR) three months postoperatively

Inclusion and Exclusion Criteria

Not all treatments are right for all patients, and not all patients who receive certain treatments are right for clinical studies. Consider the following prompts when designing your study criteria:

- Are there any contraindications to the treatment?
- Which population do you want to study?
  - Gender
  - Age range
  - Race
  - Disease state (e.g., severity of cataract, glaucoma diagnosis)

   - Baseline data range (e.g., intraocular pressure, refractive error)
   - Previous treatment history
- Is there any noncompliance risk?
- Should women who are pregnant or lactating be included?
- Is there any issue that a potential participant may have that could confound the study endpoints? For example, a patient without a potential corrected distance visual acuity of 20/25 or better after cataract surgery may not be appropriate to assess the efficacy of a new intraocular lens.

The Schedule of Visits and Follow-up Visits

For prospective and ambispective studies, you will need to decide on how many visits and in what interval each study participant will attend. Here are important visits to make sure happen:

- Informed consent. Review the consent form and answer any questions that participants may have.
- Screening. Make sure that participants meet inclusion and exclusion criteria. Collect baseline data.
- Treatment. Perform the intervention with the study device or drug on one or multiple visits.
- Follow-up. Specify how many visits are needed based on appropriate timelines to assess the safety and efficacy of the study intervention.

Assessments

Consider how you will assess safety and efficacy with your study and how often you will perform assessments. A good place to start is to create a table of visits and assessments. An example from a monofocal investigator-initiated clinical trial is shown in table 3.

Table 3: Example table of visits and assessments

Activity	Preoperative	Operative	Postoperative	Postoperative	Postoperative
	Visit 1	Visit 2	Visit 3	Visit 4	Visit 5
			1 Day	**1 Month**	**3 Months**
Informed consent	X				
Demographics	X				
General information: Medical history	X				
Surgery		X			
Manifest refraction	X			X	X
Monocular uncorrected distance VA	X		X	X	X
Monocular corrected distance VA	X			X	X
Binocular uncorrected and corrected distance VA				X	X
Binocular uncorrected and distance corrected intermediate VA (80 cm)				X	X
Binocular uncorrected and distance corrected intermediate VA (66 cm)					X
Binocular defocus curve					X
Monitor for adverse events and device deficiencies		X	X	X	X

Sample Size

How many participants (or eyes) are needed to obtain sufficient data to answer your research question? Typically, investigator-initiated trials are powered to answer the primary endpoint—but not necessarily any secondary or exploratory endpoint(s).

Many factors must be considered when deciding on an adequate sample size. A good place to start is to look at what sample sizes (and justifications) are shown in similar or otherwise comparable studies. However, I strongly encourage you to seek out the expertise of a statistician.

1. Primary endpoint. The data type for the primary endpoint affects the sample size. Some examples are patient-reported outcomes, continuous measurements, proportions, and dichotomous data.
2. Effect size. This is the expected magnitude of outcomes or differences within or between groups. Smaller effect sizes require larger sample sizes.
3. Standard deviation. The variability in measurements of your outcomes. Higher variability will require larger sample sizes to spot differences between groups
4. Alpha level. The acceptable rate of false positives for your study is generally 0.05. The smaller the alpha level, the larger the required sample size.
5. Beta level. The acceptable rate of false negatives is generally 0.2. The smaller the beta level, the larger the required sample size.

6. Study design. If your study uses paired samples (i.e., the same participant can be found in multiple groups), then the required sample size would be lower than a study that had a parallel group design. Consider the impact of other study designs.
7. Multiplicity. If your study will test multiple endpoints or include subanalyses, then you must account for the increased risk of a false positive.
8. Dropout. Adjust the final sample size by an appropriate dropout rate for your population. This number is generally 10%–20%.

Aside from the above factors to calculate a sample size, also consider the cost, logistics, and ethics of overpowered or underpowered studies.

Statistical Analysis Plan

The statistical analysis plan must be aligned with the study objectives and be carefully thought out to ensure a robust and reliable analysis. Many factors need to be considered for the plan:

1. Type of analysis. Descriptive statistics summarize the distribution, central tendency, and variability of a given dataset. Inferential statistics can be used to test your study hypothesis or make predictions about a particular population.
2. Data type. Different analyses will be needed for different types of data, such as patient-reported outcomes, continuous, ordinal, and proportions.

3. Parametric or not. Not all data collected will be normally distributed. Therefore, you should include in your plan what nonparametric methods could be used to ensure the validity of your results.
4. Number of groups. Certain types of tests, such as the popular t-test, are not necessarily appropriate for comparisons among three or more groups.
5. Missing data. If you anticipate a significant amount of missing data, consider how it will be handled. Missing data is more likely for retrospective studies, studies that use patient questionnaires, or those that have high dropout rates.
6. Subanalyses. Specify ahead of time any subanalyses that will be done and what the subgroups will be.
7. Intention to treat or per protocol. Determine whether you will analyze only the data from those participants who successfully complete the study or will include data from those who exit early.
8. Interim analysis. Describe any interim analysis, what adjustments will be made, and determine for which criteria.

Budget

After you have a detailed study design, next you should figure out how much it will cost to complete! You can engage with third parties, such as IRBs or IECs, consultants, CROs, and other vendors to get an idea of the costs to use them for your investigator-initiated study.

For your own costs, consider how many hours each staff member—including you—will need to dedicate to complete their tasks. A simple calculation would be to then multiply the hourly rate of each staff member by the anticipated number of hours and total up the costs. Keep in mind that many grants won't fund investigator travel to conferences, equipment, or investigator time. So, always be sure to read the guidelines and reach out to the funding provider for clarification.

Also consider the purchase of any consumables, equipment, or investigational devices or drugs. Many journals now also have a cost to publish (known as an open-access fee), so include them as well. The typical fee range is $3,000 to $4,500, but check a few of the journals in your field.

If you have overhead costs, include those too!

You now have all the building blocks to design a successful study. Just remember, not all types of studies will require all the parts outlined above.

SECURING GRANT FUNDING AS A PRIVATE PRACTICE

Preparing a proposal for an investigator-initiated trial can be a difficult and time-consuming task, even if you are a seasoned researcher. Here is my signature methodology to increase your chances of success.

First, consider that you must tailor the proposal to the audience. Applying for a grant from the government, academia, or from commercial partners requires a different theme, content, tone, and style of writing for each.

For example, academic grants are weighed more on the technical and scientific aspects of the project. They want to know how you will solve a particular problem. Commercial partners, however, care more about why the problem should be solved and, of course, the market size that will affect the solution!

Follow the Guidelines

Once you know the target audience, find the guidelines from the potential funding source. This document may detail the section, subsections, number of pages, and any supporting documents to submit (like a research CV). Make sure you follow all the steps and include all the required information. If you can't follow simple instructions, your application may be thrown out without much review!

Typical sections for a proposal include these items:

- The research question you want to answer
- The study design and methodology that will be used to answer the question
- The specific study objectives or endpoints
- Inclusion and exclusion criteria
- Sample size
- Statistical analysis plan
- Timeline for completion
- Publication or communication plan
- Budget

Other Things to Consider

Keep the language as simple as possible. No one can fund what they don't understand. As such, try to keep your writing concise, and define any technical terms to improve clarity. Avoid leaving out necessary information, however. You wouldn't want the application to give the impression of incompleteness.

Also be sure to proofread your work! Lots of typos and grammar mistakes can make your application look sloppy. I suggest that you have at least one other pair of eyes review your draft (using two people is even better). Having colleagues review your proposal and give specific feedback can also greatly improve your chances of success.

Add a little persuasiveness. Your job is to convince the potential partner that your proposal is the one to fund over all others under consideration for the same finite grant resources. Persuasive writing is an art form that combines both logic and emotion. You want decision-makers to understand the reasons your proposal should be funded, but you also want to leave them with a feeling that drives them to action. Ask a staff member to make suggestions as needed.

A Few Key Points to Touch On:

- Highlight yourself as the investigator! Be sure to include your accolades.
- What other studies have you been a part of? If this study is your first, say so.
- Have you published before? Spoken at conferences?

- Why is your practice perfect for answering your research question?
- What equipment, collaborators, patient population, recruitment strategies, and staff set you apart?

Once you get the first grant under your belt, it becomes easier to secure future funding. The documents and processes created for your first proposal can be modified and reused for future applications.

Here's a great example of professionals who successfully prepared a submission for a self-sponsored study. As already mentioned, Ruby and Hazel are optometrists, both working at a busy practice. They had prior experience being a part of a clinical trial sponsored by a large pharmaceutical company and wanted to secure grant funding from an ophthalmic company for their own research. However, they had never completed an investigator-initiated study before, and the applications seemed challenging, especially their first application ever! The pair worked tirelessly to understand the submission requirements of the company and simultaneously worked to streamline their grant-application process for future submissions.

They were successful in the first application, but better yet, based on how well they streamlined their application process, they were able to secure funding from the same company for not one but three clinical studies over the span of a single year! Ruby and Hazel now have the confidence and the efficient processes to apply for funding from that company as well as from other companies, academic institutions, and even government agencies.

Writing effective grant proposals is a skill that may take time to develop and may take many rejections before you get a proposal that is accepted. Don't be discouraged if you do get a rejection. Take it as a learning opportunity to improve and to increase your chances of success for next time.

CREATING A PROTOCOL THAT WILL PASS AN ETHICS REVIEW

The study protocol acts as a blueprint for conducting the study. It tells anyone who reads it the problem or gap in the literature, what research question you are trying to answer, and how you are going to answer it.

Creating the first protocol also is daunting, but once you have it done, you can use it as a template for future studies. You can start from scratch or modify an existing template. (There are plenty online to choose from.) As of the writing of this book, the International Council for Harmonisation (ICH) is also working on a Clinical Electronic Structured Harmonised Protocol that can also be a good starting point. You can find out more information on their website: https://ich.org/.

Let's walk through an example of a prospective study.

Title Page

As the name suggests, put your study title here! You will need the official title and a short version of the title. Also include the protocol version number and date.

You also need to give your protocol a unique number. It could be your grant number, if you have one. At Sengi, we prefer to use the initials of the investigator-sponsor, the year, and a two-digit unique number. For example, if Dr. Gregory House was the investigator-sponsor of a 2025 study, the protocol number could be GH-25-01.

On the title page, also be sure to add the IRB or IEC name and address, sponsor name and address, potential grant funder name and address, and your name as the investigator.

Executive Summary

This section of the protocol gives a high-level overview of the study's key details and generally all fits on one page. It includes this information:

- The objective of the study
- The study hypothesis
- Test article(s)
- Sample size
- Study population description
- Number of sites
- Study design
- Endpoints
- Duration of the study and follow-up

Introduction and Objective

Give background information about the current state of the literature and the problem that you intend to address or the gap in knowledge that you are trying to fill. How long should this section be? It should be as long as it needs to be.

Erring on the side of brevity, though, is desired with succinct writing. I recommend that introduction sections be fewer than 250 words (or one page, double-spaced).

The objective needs to clearly state the purpose of your study. It should start with something like this:

- To compare…
- To evaluate…
- To assess…

Participants

This information constitutes a very important section and will be scrutinized by the IRB or IEC. You will need to first outline the study population.

In this section, you also will describe the inclusion and exclusion criteria. Be specific with these criteria and make sure that you don't accidentally exclude portions of your target population.

Not following the inclusion or exclusion criteria is a serious issue, as is enrolling participants who don't qualify, so spend some time here getting it right.

Study Design

This section of the protocol will describe the design of your study, as the name implies. These are a few key questions you will want to answer:

- Prospective, retrospective, or ambispective?
- Single or multicenter?
- Randomization?
- Masking?

Also in this section, you can describe your endpoints. The primary endpoint is the most important measure to help answer your research question. Secondary endpoints support the primary endpoint. Exploratory endpoints are just that—exploratory. They may or may not yield any interesting results.

In addition, briefly discuss how you will minimize bias in your study. If you use randomization, you will need to outline in this section how it will be done. For example, participants could be randomized into treatment arms by simple randomization (flipping a coin).

Study Procedure

This section is also very important to the IRB or IEC because the details describe what will happen at each study visit, such as what treatment you will use and what tests participants can expect.

A useful summary to include here is a table of the visit schedule. It should show the visit numbers and visit window at a quick glance and can be a useful reference for study coordinators and technicians who will ultimately perform many of the examinations and tests for your study. An example is shown in table 4.

Table 4. Example schedule

Visit number	Visit window
1	Surgery (Day 0)
2	Postoperative day 1 (Day 1 ± 1 day)
3	Postoperative month 1 (Day 28 ± 7 days)
4	Postoperative month 3 (Day 84 ± 7 days)

In addition to the summary table, outline in detail each test that will be completed at each visit. You can use bullet points here for ease of reading. Here is an example for a baseline visit:

- Medical history
- Manifest refraction
- Corrected distance visual acuity
- Preoperative questionnaire

After outlining all the visits and the tests, now you need to describe each test in detail. You need as much detail as required so that study personnel performing the tests will do it the same way every time. For example, with visual acuity, specify the chart, distance, lighting, how to encourage participants to read harder letters, what criteria to use to stop visual acuity testing, whether to use logMAR, and whether to record to the nearest line or number of letters.

You may also briefly describe what will happen at unscheduled visits and what to do if participants exit the study prematurely or miss follow-up appointments.

Analysis Plan

I strongly recommend that you get help from a statistician to write this section. You will need to first outline if all data will be analyzed or only data from participants who completed all visits.

You also need to describe how the data will be analyzed. Will you use descriptive statistics only, or will inferential statistics be used? If so, what tests are planned to be done? You should outline the planned tests for each type of data (continuous, interval, Likert scale, parametric, nonparametric). Also, what software will be used for the analysis?

This section will also justify the sample size you selected for your study. Again, I highly recommend that you have a statistician help with it. An underpowered or overpowered study wastes resources and may have ethical concerns as well.

Boilerplate Sections

The next few parts don't change much from study to study and can be used for multiple studies once you finalize the other areas.

- Confidentiality. How will the confidentiality of study participants be protected?

- Adverse events. What constitutes an adverse event, and what should happen when a nonserious or serious adverse event occurs? How will adverse events be monitored?
- Ethical considerations. What requirements will the study comply with? Will it be registered in a clinical trials database?

Study Table

This table will be by far the most referenced object in the entire protocol. At a quick glance, it provides information about how many study visits, the visit windows for each, and what tests or treatments are to be done at each visit. Spend a disproportionate amount of time getting this information right because chances are that study personnel will only review this part of the protocol. Refer back to table 3, the example earlier in this chapter, for reference.

There you have it—a complete blueprint to create a study protocol! Putting all this together is a big undertaking, so give yourself a huge pat on the back when you're finished. All other study documents flow from here, so creating the next necessary documents is easier.

DRAFTING AN UNDERSTANDABLE INFORMED CONSENT FORM

One standard document that you will prepare for an investigator-initiated trial (unless it is a retrospective study) is the informed consent form. It is a patient-facing document that describes what the study is about, what treatments will be used, the examinations required, number of visits, risks and benefits, and patient rights. The informed consent form is designed to protect research participants from harm. Patients will need to review and sign this document before any study-related procedures can be performed. In addition, informed consent forms will need to be reviewed and approved by an IRB or IEC to ensure the rights of participants are protected.

If the informed consent form sounds like an arduous document to prepare, don't worry! This section will review the required sections and provide tips for getting it perfect for use in any investigator-initiated trial.

Because informed consent forms are required for all clinical trials (unless you are doing a retrospective study), many templates are available online. Most IRB or IECs will also have their own template that I encourage you to use. If you want a general place to start, check out these forms from the WHO.[8] As you modify any template, keep in mind that you want the writing to be kept at a reading level no higher than eighth grade. (Document-preparation services within software, such as MS Word, allow you to view the reading level.)

The International Council for Harmonisation (ICH) released recommendations for the informed consent in ICH Good

8 "Research Ethics Review Committee (ERC)," World Health Organization, accessed August 29, 2025, https://www.who.int/groups/research-ethics-review-committee/guidelines-on-submitting-research-proposals-for-ethics-review/templates-for-informed-consent-forms.

Clinical Practice (GCP) E6(R3).[9] If you read the document—and I encourage you to—all those points can seem very overwhelming. However, if you grab a template, you will generally see all this information broken down by three overarching sections with subsections. The first section is simply basic information, which includes the study title, purpose of the research, investigator name and contact information, and an invitation to enroll in your research study.

The next section gets more detailed. There, you need to outline how the study will be conducted—namely, what intervention(s) is planned, how many visits are required, what will happen at each of those visits, the length of the study, the number of participants, risks and benefits of participation, and any reimbursement to the participants.

Last, you'll provide the details about how confidentiality will be maintained, who might have access to participant data, what to do in case of emergency, legal rights, whom to contact during the study, how to leave the study, and finally a signature page for both the participant and the staff member who explained the informed consent document.

One final tip is to be as concise as possible and to write with plain language. Remember that a participant has to read and understand the form, so it is better to keep the length down and the comprehension up.

9 *ICH Harmonised Guideline: Good Clinical Practice (GCP) E6(R3)*, International Council for Harmonisation for Better Health, May 19, 2023, https://database.ich.org/sites/default/files/ICH_E6%28R3%29_DraftGuideline_2023_0519.pdf.

Drafting an informed consent form is a lot easier when you start with a template, modifying it for your particular study and your site. Once you have done one, modifying the form continues to become a lot easier for future studies.

AVOID DELAYS: KEEP YOUR DOCUMENTS UPDATED

As part of the IRB or IEC submission process, you will need to submit a CV, a copy of your medical license, and proof of human subjects protection and good clinical practice training. Overlooking those documents can unnecessarily delay approvals.

For example, Jasper didn't list anywhere on his CV that he had prior clinical trial experience. The IRB or IEC delayed the submission until the issue was rectified, costing a one-week delay.

Keeping all essential investigator documents up to date will ensure an efficient start-up process and clinical trial success. Here are a few tips to make the IRB or IEC's review of your documents easier.

Your CV should, of course, list your education and job experience. However, you should have a summary to highlight your clinical research expertise, wherein you list all studies that you have been a part of and your role in them. Keep this information up to date as well. Also be sure to highlight if you have credentials in clinical research (such as through the Association of Clinical Research Professionals, https://acrpnet.org/) as well as any training that you have completed, such as GCP. Overall, make your CV concise, chronological, and easy to review.

A digital copy of your medical license will also be required for review by the IRB or IEC simply to check that you are legally allowed to practice medicine. Where some investigators cause unnecessary delays is by forgetting to make a fresh copy every time their license is renewed. I recommend setting a calendar reminder for yourself to create a digital copy at the same regular interval that your license renews and keep the image of your updated license where you can easily locate it for future studies.

Proof of GCP training will also be reviewed by the IRB or IEC. GCP is an internationally recognized standard, ensuring that you are familiar with protecting patient rights and adhering to regulatory standards, data integrity, etc. Although the training can be time-consuming, it is a mistake to think of it as just a box to tick. Don't rush through the training. Following GCP guidelines is fundamental to a successful clinical trial.

Many accredited organizations provide GCP training. One of the most well-known is Collaborative Institutional Training Initiative (CITI, https://about.citiprogram.org/). Some other options are available through the National Institutes of Health (https://www.nih.gov/) and also likely through the IRB or IEC that you selected. Whichever provider you choose, make sure that they are accredited and that your certificate has your name, course completion date, the name of the provider, and an expiration date (if there is one). If there is an expiration date, add a calendar reminder for yourself to update the requirements before the expiration date to avoid unnecessary study delays.

Note that only investigators are required to submit proof of GCP training to the IRB or IEC for investigator-initiated studies, but all study staff who will be involved in the clinical trial should also complete human subjects protection and GCP training to ensure compliance.

Keeping investigator documents in order can seem like a burden, but it really is a core part of doing clinical research. Staying on top of any administrative task ensures high-quality, ethical research that ultimately creates an impact in eye care.

NAVIGATING ETHICS SUBMISSIONS FOR FASTER APPROVALS

The principles of the LENS Launch with Focus step encompass the IRB or IEC process as well. All clinical trials need ethical oversight. Each IRB or IEC will have its own process for submitting documents and even specific templates that they want followed by eye-care professionals. To create efficiency in your research, the best practice is to find one IRB or IEC to use and stick with them, unless you have good reason to change. By sticking with the same IRB or IEC, you then have templates and processes that can be reused for future studies.

The study protocol created earlier is invaluable during the IRB or IEC submission process. Not only is the protocol a required document to submit, but also the IRB or IEC will have a series of forms that need to be completed and submitted along with it. The different sections of the protocol can be repurposed for these submission forms, streamlining this process. For non-retrospective studies, you will generally be required to submit an informed consent form. Each IRB or IEC has its general template that I recommend to use. However, the study protocol can be re-purposed and used again to fill in the required sections.

A quick note about private versus institutional IRBs or IECs—private IRBs or IECs are for-profit companies that review clinical studies and make sure they are compliant with all applicable regulations. Institutional IRBs or IECs do the same thing, but they are generally affiliated with a hospital or university.

Without question, using a private IRB or IEC is best if you can. Why? Because such reviews are at the core of their function. With an institutional IRB or IEC, members are generally hospital or university staff, whose core responsibilities are not to review studies but to see patients and to teach. As such, a private IRB will issue an approval much more quickly than an institutional IRB.

Here is a perfect example of the benefits of using a private IRB.

Julia aimed to conduct an investigator-initiated trial that was more involved than average. She wanted to include randomization, multiple arms, and masking. Using the principles of Launch with Focus, Julia was able to get the necessary documents in front of a private IRB within one week and had approval after another one and a half weeks—for a total of just two and a half weeks!

Contrast this with another project—one by Jacob, who wanted to conduct a similar investigator-initiated trial—with two arms, randomization, and masking. However, he chose an institutional IRB or IEC for review. The institutional IRB or IEC took six months to respond with its initial comments! Such a lengthy turnaround is ridiculously slow—so slow, in fact, that the grant funder pulled their support over the delay.

Keep in mind that nonretrospective trials should also be registered in a clinical trials database, such as clinicaltrials.gov, prior to enrollment of the first patient, or within 30 days of the first patient being enrolled. Here, too, the protocol can be repurposed to fill in the required sections. For greater efficiency, consider completing the IRB or IEC submission forms and registration in a clinical trials database in parallel since they don't depend on each other. In fact, the registration should be completed in advance of any participants being enrolled. Consider the following consequence of ignoring this start-up step.

Many medical journals now require registration of a clinical trial in a clinical trials registry, such as clinicaltrials.gov, for any article that is published. Thankfully, registries like clinicaltrials.gov don't charge a fee. Keep in mind that if this step is skipped, your manuscript could be rejected even before peer review.

That consequence happened to Lucas, who had written up a manuscript for publication from the results of his investigator-initiated trial. It was a prospective study of a new medical device. However, the editor came back with a shocking decision of rejection before even sending the manuscript for peer review, solely based on the fact that the study was not registered in a clinical trials database.

Lucas was able to successfully appeal the decision, and his paper was eventually accepted and published, but be aware that its publication was an exception, not the rule, and the decision remains at the discretion of the editor.

Another example of this happened to Veronica, who submitted a manuscript based on the results of a retrospective investigator-initiated study, despite such studies not even being required to be registered. Yet, her manuscript still was flagged and rejected by the automated submission system.

MAKE AN IMPACT

- On one page, roughly sketch out your study design, including the research question, intervention, study population, and key endpoints.
- Create a folder and store within it all your investigator documents.
- Look into one source for grant funding: government, medical society, or company.
- Identify the IRB or IEC that you would use for your study's approval.
- Download protocol and informed consent templates and review the sections.

CHAPTER 5: ENROLL WITH CONFIDENCE

RECRUITMENT AND RETENTION KEYS

The LENS Enroll with Confidence step is your ability to quickly recruit patients and have all or almost all of them complete every follow-up visit.

Since the purpose of a clinical trial is to collect data and test a hypothesis, if you can't recruit patients, you can't collect data. If recruited patients don't attend all visits, then the quality of your data suffers and calls into question the validity of your results.

Getting the desired numbers of patients to become enrolled in the study needs to be completed in a timely manner. Not only will firm recruitment help to keep costs down, as the project will be completed much quicker, but it also can increase the number of clinical trials that your practice can do per year.

Likewise, getting enrolled participants to complete all visits is equally as important as recruitment. If 100 participants are recruited for your trial, but only 60 complete the final visit and give you the crucial pieces of data that are needed to answer the research question, then the study is a failure and a waste of time, money, and resources.

If you can reliably recruit and retain participants in clinical trials, then you will complete trials on time, and more importantly, on budget. The reputation you establish from such success can assure sponsors so that they will want to work with you.

A STUDY COORDINATOR IS VITAL TO RECRUITMENT AND RETENTION

Having the right research team will make or break a clinical trial. Here, I provide an example of how your efforts can quickly go bad if your team is not in order.

Lucy was an investigator on a multicenter clinical trial. At the start of the trial, everything was going well. Patients were being recruited, then retained during follow-up, and the data was being collected at a steady pace. However, all the progress fell apart when the study coordinator left the site. Lucy didn't see the need to have a dedicated coordinator for the study anymore and instead relied on untrained staff themselves to fill in ad hoc.

Everything just fell apart. New participants were not being recruited, patients who had been attending follow-up visits suddenly stopped coming, and the data that was once being generated like a fire hose became a trickle. The study site was eventually closed down, with much of the data unusable. Moreover, the site's reputation suffered significantly, leading to lost opportunities of getting involved in other studies.

What the example highlights is the importance of having a research team in place. Your team will be the backbone of a successful clinical trial, ensuring efficiency, quality, regulatory compliance, and ultimately, better patient care.

As that background highlights, the importance of a dedicated study coordinator cannot be overstated. Their responsibilities are generally to manage the day-to-day operations of a study, such as patient recruitment, scheduling follow-up visits, and data collection. Aside from the principal investigator, the study coordinator role is of the highest importance if you want to have a successful clinical trial and make an impact in eye care. The principal investigator leads the trial and often performs all the medical interventions, but the study coordinator is the patient-facing part of the whole operation. Without somebody managing trial operations, as Lucy's example illustrates, the whole trial falls apart.

THE KEY ATTRIBUTES FOR AN ALL-STAR STUDY COORDINATOR

1. A good candidate would have (*a*) knowledge and prior experience in clinical trials, ideally in eye care, (*b*) familiarity with regulatory requirements, such as good clinical practice and knowledge of IRBs or IECs, and (*c*) excellent organizational and time-management skills.

2. Candidates need to be effective communicators, as they will interact directly with patients and other study team member on a regular basis.
3. Problem-solving skills also are an asset as clinical research can come with many unexpected challenges that need to be managed.
4. Attention to detail is needed to ensure data accuracy and to catch errors before they become bigger problems.
5. Other aspects of the role can be learned, such as an EDC system if you are using one.

Finding the right study coordinator can be tricky, but without this key role, any clinical trial can completely fall apart and lead to wasted resources and a poor reputation for your practice. However, if you can hire a candidate with experience, organization, problem-solving skills, and attention to detail, then you will dramatically increase your chances of a successful clinical trial. The right person in that position will ultimately lead to more efficient recruitment, higher retention, and better data.

START BY RECRUITING YOUR OWN PATIENTS

The best place to look for participants for an investigator-initiated clinical trial is with your internal patient population. You undoubtedly have a steady flow of patients visiting your practice. It is not that much extra effort to let them know they likely are a good candidate for a clinical trial that you are running.

Many eye-care professionals make the mistake of thinking that their patients won't be interested. I think such hesitancy comes from a lack of understanding of how a study can augment patient care. An ongoing trial may have new treatment available that is perfect for your patients, and it's potentially inaccessible unless they are in a study. That outcome makes the trial an additional care option for patients. Research doesn't have to be separate from patient care—both can work together.

To begin recruiting from your own patient population, you can start by having staff look through your electronic health records. Identify patients who could benefit from your study by checking to see who might be eligible against the inclusion and exclusion criteria of the study. With a list of potential candidates in hand, staff can systematically reach out to potential participants about their interest. Patients coming in for routine visits can also be flagged and approached to see if they want to participate.

Successfully integrating internal recruitment will take some work. First, frontline staff will need to be trained to identify potential candidates and approach them to be in the study. Make sure everyone has a thorough understanding of the informed consent process. It is actually much easier to have a point person for your studies who identifies, screens, and follows up with potential participants in order to create a seamless workflow. As discussed earlier, a study coordinator is crucial to clinical trial success. They take care of the managing the day-to-day operations! Regular contact from the staff with participants will increase retention as well.

Technology can also be of great help. Once your study has been approved by the IRB or IEC, text messages and email campaigns can significantly boost recruitment compared to just waiting for eligible patients to walk through the front door.

Technology can also eliminate the need for patients to come into the clinic at all!

Let's look at an example.

Herbert was conducting a multicenter investigator-initiated trial where no patients had an in-person visit. They were identified via their electronic health records, then called on the phone. Consent was done over the phone or video chat, and their signature was obtained via an electronic document application. Then, the patients were sent an online survey to complete. Easy peasy!

Although recruiting patients is vital, it doesn't have to be overly complicated. Generally, you can achieve most or all of your target enrollment from your own patient population. Moreover, by integrating research into your patient care, you can offer additional benefits to them as well as gain the speed and efficiency of recruitment for yourself. Go ahead and start identifying and engaging with your patients today!

EXPAND YOUR RECRUITMENT POOL

In the last section, we covered how your own patient population is the best place to start to recruit patients. However, using your internal resources does have its limits. To ensure clinical trial success, you can expand the recruitment pool by partnering with local clinics.

The following scenario illustrates that exact issue. Aria is an eye-care professional at a thriving practice, but her investigator-initiated trial was slow on recruitment. She had overestimated the number of potential participants from her own patient population who would qualify based on the inclusion and exclusion criteria of the study. The study was in danger of being stopped early without hitting the necessary sample size for a meaningful analysis.

By partnering with other eye-care professionals in the area, however, Aria was able to get the necessary referrals to hit the recruitment target and finish on time. The study was completed successfully and published in a medical journal. Actually, it was so successful that it spawned a follow-up study with the same grant provider!

You might be thinking that other clinics wouldn't dream of referring their patients because you are their competition. This notion is a mistake. In fact, other clinics may lack the specialized care required for some of their patients, so your clinical trial could be a great opportunity to treat their patients. Other eye-care professionals and even primary care physicians may be able to refer the perfect candidates to you. That strategy is especially true for these providers:

- Eye-care professionals of another specialty
- Those who don't conduct research
- Those who treat early-stage conditions
- Those who currently refer patients to you
- Primary care physicians who are managing current ocular conditions

Remember (and remind your colleagues) that you are not taking their patients but simply offering advanced-treatment options and comanaged care. Be sure to reciprocate when possible.

If you want referrals, you need to make it super simple for others to give them to you. Again, having a dedicated study coordinator who can be a point of contact for referring doctors can make things a lot easier. The study coordinator can also work with referring doctors to ensure that only eligible patients for your current study are referred, saving everyone's time. The study coordinator can also do regular follow-ups to keep referring doctors in the loop and to keep the referral pipeline active.

Connecting with your colleagues for referrals can be as simple as direct outreach. Have your staff pick up the phone and call around, then send personalized emails as a follow-up. In chapter 7, we will discuss how to share your results to position you and your practice as a recognized researcher and key opinion leader, which will attract referrals. Attending smaller, local eye-care conferences can also be a great way to connect with potential collaborators.

The option of getting referrals from local clinics is one of the most often-overlooked areas of recruitment and can lead to clinical trial failure. An effective strategy to accelerate recruitment is by establishing and maintaining relationships with referring doctors. Now, get out there and build your network!

USE STRATEGIC MARKETING TO BOOST RECRUITMENT

For larger studies, where you need to recruit many participants, or for studies with narrower inclusion and exclusion criteria that limit the potential study population, you can still hit your recruitment numbers using marketing.

Juan was struggling to recruit for his investigator-initiated study with just his own patient population because the inclusion and exclusion criteria had narrowed down his pool of potential participants. In addition, many local colleagues who normally refer patients did not have a large pool of candidates either. Juan decided to create a radio ad to market the study to a wider audience. Indeed, the ad worked, and he was able to complete enrollment on time and keep the grant funder happy!

The strategic deployment of marketing as part of your overall clinical trial recruitment strategy can give you the boost you need to make it over the finish line. One of the biggest obstacles to overcome is that many eligible participants are completely unaware that you are conducting a clinical study. An effective marketing strategy can reach more people (faster) than in-office visits with your own patients.

The first avenue to explore is traditional media, especially if you are looking to recruit from older demographics. Consider radio (as in Juan's example), print ads in local newspapers, and flyers. Second, you can leverage social media to reach more potential candidates. It can be as simple as creating a post about the study and paying a service to get it in front of more eyeballs. Social media platforms also allow for digital ads targeted by age, location, and interests so that you can focus on and reach more of the right candidates. Finally, a more passive approach could be to provide information about your ongoing studies on your practice website if you are getting a reasonable amount of web traffic.

With any approach, you want to make sure you use clear messaging about the study and have received IRB or IEC approval of any marketing materials before use. The most effective ads avoid misleading claims, are transparent about the risks and benefits of participation, use plain language, and may address common fears and misinformation. Here is an example of effective digital ad copy:[10]

"Do you have cataract surgery coming up? You may be eligible to participate in a clinical trial evaluating a new intraocular lens that is designed to provide clear vision after surgery. Adults who will undergo cataract surgery in both eyes and meet basic health criteria can join. The study involves three visits over three months with experienced ophthalmologists, and you will be compensated $100 per study visit. Call [phone number] for details!"

Adding marketing to your recruitment efforts can effectively build a sustainable research pipeline for current and future studies, ensuring that you always meet your enrollment targets. You can start by implementing one new marketing strategy, then build from there. Use the success of your marketing choice(s) to determine which service gets the best result, but don't limit yourself unnecessarily.

10 More templates are available from https://sengiclinical.com/eyedeatoimpact.

OFFER PROPER COMPENSATION

A quick note about incentives in investigator-initiated clinical trials—a delicate balance exists between compensating study participants for their time and participation and the undue influence from overly high incentives. Any reputable IRB or IEC will help you navigate this—and let you know if your compensation conflicts with ethical standards—but you can save time and get approval faster by following these tips.

First, as discussed in the previous section, many different ways are available to compensate patients for their participation, including these:

- Financial incentives such as a fee paid per visit
- Support for travel such as transportation, parking, lodging, and food
- Health care support, such as free screenings, diagnostic tests, and study treatment and follow-up care

One common mistake that new investigators make is to provide up front the total amount of compensation for the entire study, rather than a set amount for each completed visit. I'm sure you can see how that allowance can cause some patients to drop out early.

Another common mistake, as alluded to before, is not offering enough incentive. That misstep generally stems from an investigator's lack of empathy for the burden placed on patients to participate in the study. Put yourself in the shoes of a study participant who has to take significant time out of their busy life to join the study—or the caregiver who drives them. A paltry sum is not going to encourage participation and can even be insulting.

On the flip side, it is also a mistake to overly compensate patients for participation, and this can be flagged by the IRB or IEC as potential coercion. Offering a large dollar amount for participation can be really attractive to a low-income patient and can cloud their judgment to the perceived risks of the study. One rule of thumb is to think of incentives as **compensation** rather than a **reward**. I typically see compensation between $150 to $300 per participant for investigator-initiated trials in eye care.

Offering incentives for participation in your investigator-initiated clinical trial should be a win-win for yourself and your patients if done correctly. They get compensated for their time and participation, and you can accelerate your recruitment efforts and maintain a low-dropout rate.

KEEP PARTICIPANTS ENGAGED TO REDUCE DROPOUTS

Recruiting patients into a study can be exciting, especially when you know they can benefit from the treatment. However, recruiting patients into the study is only half the battle. The other half is keeping them in the study. When patients drop out from your study, not only do you lose any data after that point, but you also typically reduce your final sample size overall.

IRBs and IECs grant approval to recruit a certain number of patients. When someone joins your study but then leaves (also known as a dropout), they still count toward your approved number of patients allowed. Sample-size calculations often include a 10%–15% buffer to account for unexpected dropout. However, if your studies have overly high dropout rates, the outcome adversely affects timelines and data integrity.

Patients drop out for all sorts of reasons—some actually are outside your control—but you want to make sure to watch out for some of the top issues so that you don't unnecessarily and adversely affect the study's retention requirements.

One of the top reasons is that the study requirements are simply too burdensome. As a patient, I was involved in a study that required participants to remain at the study site without leaving the building for an entire day, starting early in the morning and finishing sometime in the evening after dinner. The study did reduce that burden of participating by monetary compensation, and the sponsor did provide meals throughout the day. I was a graduate student and worked in the same building, so that location made it easier for me. But for prospects whose work was at another location, the mandate would have been quite cumbersome and therefore tougher to accept.

My advice is to think like a study participant and try to reduce the burden as much as possible. Eliminate some unnecessary exams or visits if you can. You can also compensate for burdens with money, paid accommodations, food, travel, and childcare.

Patients may also feel disconnected and drop out if there is a lack of communication from study staff. People are busy and have constantly changing motivations. If study staff are not regularly checking in with participants and reminding them of their upcoming appointments, they may lose interest or forget about the study entirely.

Unrealistic expectations are also a significant cause of early dropout. It is very important to completely inform participants during screening about what the study involves, the benefits, the potential adverse events, and be realistic about the expected outcomes after treatment. If not, patients may be surprised, feel misled, and choose to drop out.

Last, another key area where you can be proactive in reducing participant dropout is in nailing your clinical operations. Be sure all site staff are courteous, listen to concerns, and connect with participants. Keep a focus on reduced wait times and on an overall desirable flow of each study visit. Participants will get frustrated by long wait times, mismanagement, and poor bedside manner—and ultimately not come back for follow-up visits.

To ensure a high-retention rate in your studies, practice clear communication from the start, make participation as easy as possible, regularly engage with all participants, and make every interaction with study participants a positive experience.

MAKE AN IMPACT

- Decide whether a staff member can take on the role of study coordinator or whether you need to expand your team.

- Do a rough search through your own electronic medical records to get an idea of how big a population you have available from which to recruit.
- Identify 2–3 other eye-care practices where you already get or could get referrals for your study.
- Consider whether you will need marketing efforts to meet enrollment targets.

CHAPTER 6:
NOTICE THE INSIGHTS

REVEALING THE RESEARCH QUESTION

The LENS Notice the Insights step means to have data diligence and collect valid and useful data that will answer the research question. It encompasses many parts and starts with figuring out which pieces of data are critical to achieving the study objective(s). You certainly want to collect sufficient data for your study—otherwise, what is the point of conducting a trial if you don't collect enough data to answer the research question? However, don't fall into the other trap of collecting reams of unnecessary data, because you will waste resources not only on collecting it but also on trying to analyze or filter through it.

It is also important to then make sure that each piece of data follows ALCOA+, which stands for attributable, legible, contemporaneous, original, accurate, complete, consistent, enduring, and available. Put simply, each piece of data gathered meets these criteria:

- The data is linked to who collected it.
- You can easily read and understand it.
- It was recorded as soon as possible.
- It was not transcribed from another source.
- The data is free of errors, deletions, or missing data.
- The record has clear date and time stamps.
- The format preserves integrity, quality, and readability.

If you don't know who collected the data, you can't ask clarification questions. If you can't read the data, it is meaningless. If you don't immediately record the data, it may become lost. If you transcribe data, errors can develop. Error-prone data can lead to false conclusions. Data that has been destroyed by water damage or corrupted hard drives cannot be recovered for analysis, dissemination, or review by regulatory authorities. Create and keep a duplicate of your study's essential components in a protected area.

If you are diligent with your data, then you will have quality data and can confidently answer any research question. Not only will your diligence increase the impact you will have in eye care, but it will also boost your reputation as a go-to practice for clinical trials.

HOW TO DECIDE WHAT DATA TO COLLECT—AND WHAT TO IGNORE

The LENS Notice the Insights step begins with deciding what data to collect. You can get drawn off the path and go down deep rabbit holes if you are not careful. Are you thinking that data is easy to collect, so why not collect data on everything?

"Hair color, favorite food, cat or dog at home? Should I just explore to see if any of these have an impact on ocular care?" I have seen extraneous inquiries happen, though not to such an extreme. Inexperienced investigators tend to want to check dozens of factors to see if any has an impact on one of the study endpoints. But that approach is wrong.

First of all, you don't want to overburden patients with a lot of unnecessary tests or lengthy questionnaires. It is already time-consuming enough for patients to take time out of their day for study visits. Seeking to collect more data than necessary is not respectful of their time and, worse, risks your patients not returning to follow-up visits. Watch out also for possible ethical concerns about collecting data in a shotgun approach rather than being precise. An IRB or IEC may take issue with a study design that aims to collect data not central to answering the research question.

Second, when you're ready to do your analysis, you will likely find a lot of wasted time and resources by looking at 20 different comparisons instead of the two or three that actually matter. Try to focus on collecting data that strictly helps answer your research question.

Furthermore, including unnecessary parameters could inflate the data error rates. A type 1 error is a false positive, meaning that you reject the null hypothesis when it is true, while a type 2 error is failing to reject the null hypothesis when it is false, or a false negative. Each additional statistical test increases the probability of a false positive from 5% (from the standard alpha = 0.05) to 23% after five tests, and 40% after 10 tests. A visual example is shown in figure 1.

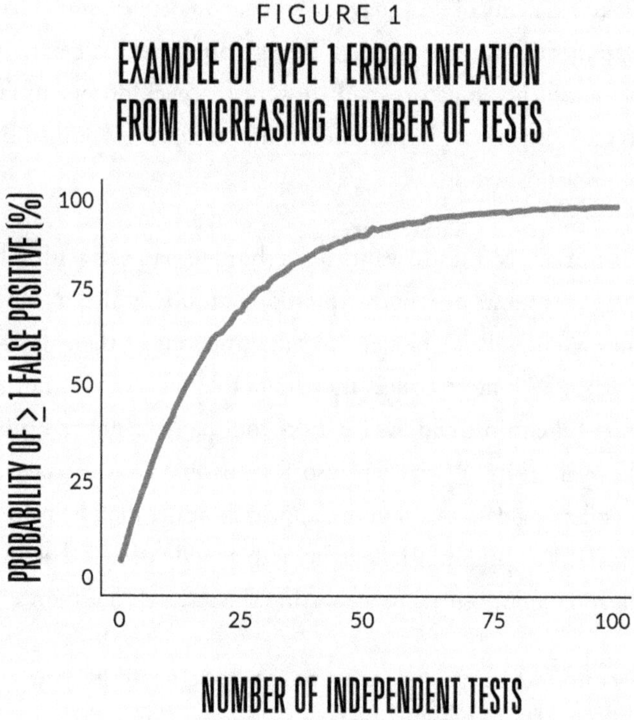

Figure 1: Example of type 1 error inflation from increasing number of tests

Finally, even if you had the resources to collect an enormous amount of data and could control for any inflated type 1 error rate, the excess data would ultimately muddle your messaging about your study. To have an impact in eye care, the goal is to be on stage speaking about your research at conferences and publishing the results in a medical journal. Your messaging will be lost if you try to report too many endpoints. Consider that the human attention span is finite and that we only remember a few main takeaways from any given presentation or journal article. Therefore, you want to focus your efforts on only investigating and looking at relevant endpoints, not going on a fishing expedition looking to find an interesting correlation.

The best way to find out what data to collect is to review the literature, find studies similar to yours, and see what they reported. If there is no paper very similar or close to yours, piece together the specifics from a few different sources. You want to see what demographic and baseline data are relevant to report, as well as typical study endpoints. Armed with that knowledge, you are ready to move on and decide not only what to collect but also **how** to actually collect it.

Here's a very interesting client experience to guide your choice of data selection.

William was conducting a retrospective investigator-initiated trial. The purpose of the study was to assess a power-calculation formula for accuracy in predicting the final refractive error in eyes implanted with a new intraocular lens. In a retrospective study, however, there's no real limit to what data you can collect, so William decided to add in an exploratory endpoint to consider another power-calculation formula in the same study. His foresight turned out to be a great decision, as the data seemed to show that one formula performed better than another in a subset of the patient population. However, because the other formula was added as an exploratory endpoint, William could not definitively show that it was a better predictor in this data subset.

What his insight did accomplish, though, was getting a large medical device company interested in a follow-up study to see for certain which formula was more accurate. The company provided full grant funding for another investigator-initiated trial. In the follow-up study, William indeed found strong evidence that one formula outperformed the other for a given patient subset. He published that insight in a medical journal, and his research now affects patient care worldwide.

It just goes to show that you never know what you are going to discover when conducting a clinical trial. Therefore, when considering what data to collect, also consider future studies. Are there standard clinical-care measurements that you are already doing that could be systematically recorded and used to support future retrospective studies?

Deciding what data to collect is a balancing act. A seemingly insignificant exploratory endpoint can end up stealing the show and lead to more opportunities for collaboration, but too much data can cloud your research results and cancel your effort to obtain results worthy of being published and acknowledged.

COLLECTING GOOD DATA REQUIRES THE RIGHT TOOLS

The next step under Notice the Insights is deciding how to collect data. It may seem trivial, but so many things can go wrong if you don't plan this step out properly. Let me give you an example.

Shelly was a study coordinator at a busy practice. She had very little training and was pulled into the study out of desperation when the previous study coordinator left. Unfortunately, that study coordinator did not properly hand off the study to Shelly or train her well, and she was left unaware of the specific worksheets that needed to be filled in to record visual acuity in clinical trials.

The worksheets are helpful guides and served as a record so that the visual acuities could be reviewed later if questions arose. Because she didn't know about the worksheets, Shelly did not use them, and being poorly trained, she recorded visual acuities wrong. Since such worksheets were unavailable to show how the visual acuities were measured, possible corrections could not be made, and the data was lost for many participants.

Having the right tools in place and the knowledge of how to use them make a big difference. That ability is the whole idea behind CRFs, which are standardized worksheets to record relevant data for the trial. They can be as simple as paper forms (as in Shelly's example) or electronic systems. Regardless of the format, all should contain key features, like these:

- Easily understood and completed
- Inclusive of dates and participant numbers attributable to every piece of data
- Confidential and securely stored in a place that minimizes data loss

In my 10-plus years in clinical research, I have seen some bad ways to record data. Let me share some tasks that you should **not** do if you want clinical trial success:

- Write data with no context (e.g., such as "20"; 20 what?)
- Mix data from multiple participants (i.e., being unable to know what data belongs to which participant)
- Have multiple pages of data but no dates (i.e., rendering the record indistinguishable from baseline versus follow-up visits)
- Throw away the original copies of data
- Forget to record a key endpoint for many participants
- Write down data illegibly
- Scribble over old data with new data, making both impossible to discern

Spend a good amount of time to ensure the integrity and quality of the data collected if you want to have clinical trial success. Here are some essential tips to help you improve your data collection:

- Provide clear instructions on how to fill out the form.
- Avoid duplication of data and unwanted details.
- Be generous with white space to allow for ease of use and viewing.
- Use consistent formatting throughout.
- Avoid ambiguous text responses. Instead, use predetermined answers (yes/no, mild/moderate/severe).
- Use proper format for entries that are numbers. Specify decimal places, if relevant.
- Use checkboxes to avoid over circling answers.

- Avoid complicated calculations that study staff need to complete during the patient visits. Leave those tasks to data analysis later.
- Record the participant ID, date, and form version on every page.

I posted a sample template that you can download at https://sengiclinical.com/eyedeatoimpact.

If you decide to use an electronic program for data capture (also known as an EDC system), a lot of those design tips will already be a part of the software. In addition, such software contains many other useful features, such as automatic data verification to minimize data-entry errors (and no issues trying to read illegible handwriting!), audit trails, and administrative burdens. Be aware that many modern systems come at an enormous cost (US$2,000+ per month) and may be more cost-effective for larger multisite investigator-initiated trials. More affordable options are available, however, many universities and hospitals host the EDC system REDCap on their own servers, which researchers at those institutions could access. At Sengi, we host EDC systems on our own server, which clients can access. Aside from cost, beware of the typically steep learning curve to start using these systems, so it may also be more time efficient to stick with paper forms for a single site and study.

A CAUTIONARY TALE ABOUT OVERCOMPLICATING TRIALS

Make the aspects of your study and the methods you choose as clear as possible for yourself and for your patients because the simplicity will benefit both. Here's an example of the difficulty involved in the electronic approach to data capture.

Frank was conducting a clinical trial in eye care with about 35 patients. The trial was started by using paper forms of the case report. By using the proper procedures previously discussed here, paper forms don't present a problem and are very cost-effective for a small(er) single-site trial. However, as previously mentioned, using an electronic form(s) for case reports does have advantages, such as fewer data-entry errors.

To chase the advantages of an electronic system and to transition from paper, Frank hired a company that specialized in EDC systems part way through the trial. The transition took months, however, due to a lot of back-and-forth about the various features of the electronic system and the data being captured. In the end, the electronic system became so bloated that the transition was abandoned, and Frank stuck with the paper CRFs. His pursuit of an electronic format had cost thousands of dollars and many hours of wasted time.

The point of the story is to reveal the many shiny objects in clinical research that can distract you—such as EDC systems, electronic ways of collecting patient-reported outcomes, and automatic summaries of data in real time. Such features have their place for large multisite clinical trials, but caution is needed when trying to use them for single-site investigator-initiated studies. Professionals must weigh the complexity and cost, and paper forms might be the best path forward.

BEST PRACTICES FOR MEANINGFUL PATIENT-REPORTED OUTCOMES

Patient-reported outcomes (PROs) can be immensely useful pieces of data to collect. They provide a perspective beyond simple visual acuity or intraocular pressure. PROs reveal the patient perspective, which answers great questions like these:

- Do patients think the treatment was effective?
- Did they experience drawbacks beyond what was measured?
- Would they have the same treatment again if they could go back in time?
- Is the drug or device something that they would recommend to friends and family after having used it?

Answers to such questions provide insights that study staff might otherwise miss.

PROs can be very helpful, but when you decide to use them, the first question to address is "Which one?"

In eye care, various questionnaires are used and published in clinical studies. How do you know which one to use? My recommendation would be to find a study (or multiple studies) similar to yours and see what those researchers used. Avoid the temptation to create your own unless there are no viable alternatives. Using PROs that are gathered using the same format makes comparison easier between studies. Not only do you get that benefit, but using your own questionnaire when other options exist—especially validated ones—degrades the impact of your research. It's also wasted effort.

When comparing different questionnaires, give extra points to ones that are validated, especially those used in pivotal trials for regulatory approval. A note of caution—check whether the questionnaire is under copyright protection, and if it is, reach out to the copyright holder well ahead of time for permission to use it or ask how to protect the copyright. How far ahead? Think in the study design phase.

Here's one scenario to illustrate potential complications.

Howard was working on a study where the copyright holder originally wanted tens of thousands of dollars to use their questionnaire! Luckily, he was able to convey the academic nature of the study and pay only a nominal fee, but not all copyright holders will be as reasonable. Moreover, you don't want to have to go back to a collaborator or grant funder and change the study design because of issues with getting approval to use a protected instrument. Don't risk unnecessary delays, which would put the project at risk of being canceled at the last minute.

If you do decide to create a questionnaire from scratch, consider these tips:

- Keep the language concise and at a third-grade reading level to enhance comprehension.
- Craft the language carefully to avoid bias in responses.
- Encourage participants to answer fully and truthfully, noting that there are no wrong answers.

Most PROs are typically gathered on paper, but you can take the tool a step further by using electronic PROs. That format is especially useful in ambispective studies, where participants have already had the treatment and just some follow-up data needs to be collected. Rather than bringing patients into your practice, you can save them time—and study resources—by using e-consent and ePROs. Keep in mind that some patients might need help with instructions on using those methods.

Finally, for any PRO measurement, carefully consider the timing. In order to show treatment benefit, you may need to have participants provide answers **before and after** treatment. In that case, consider the participants' availability and whether the PRO is needed at any particular visit. For example, some validated questionnaires in eye care are over 30 questions long! Try to make the task as convenient as possible and state whether participants could complete it at only the final visit of the study.

A well-executed collection of PROs greatly enhances success for investigator-initiated trials. By following the aforementioned best practices, you will ensure a lasting impact in eye care.

DATA ANALYSIS THAT ACTUALLY ANSWERS THE RESEARCH QUESTION

Now that you have decided on what data to collect and how to do it, the next step in Notice the Insights is to analyze the data. This step is crucial, as the goal is to finally answer the research question!

- Is treatment A effective and safe?
- Does treatment B perform better than treatment C?

There are definitely right and wrong ways to analyze data, so the use of a biostatistician for this detailed task is highly recommended. If you conduct the wrong statistical test, you will get the wrong answer. Remember—garbage in, garbage out. Only the right test will properly answer the research question. I will provide a few general conditions to avoid if you wish to try to analyze on your own.

The first pitfall to avoid is improperly summarizing data. When collecting data that consists of numbers, the tendency is to want to summarize everything as an average (mean value), but it's not always the most appropriate way to summarize data.

An example of this misuse would be the Patient-Reported Outcomes with LASIK Symptoms and Satisfaction (PROWL-SS) questionnaire, which can be summarized using mean values, but that's not the case with the Assessment of IntraOcular Lens Implant Symptoms (AIOLIS) questionnaire. Data summaries instead should provide the percentages of participants' responses on each question.

The next pitfall to avoid is using a statistical test without validating the assumptions that go into it. A classic example is the t-test. Before using it, you need to check that the data are continuous, randomly sampled, and normally distributed and that the variance in each group is approximately the same. If these assumptions are violated, such as the data are not normally distributed, then you should use a different test, such as the Mann-Whitney U test.

Finally, avoid chasing statistical significance. A lot of novice researchers get tempted into thinking that if the results do not show statistical significance, then the study is a failure and no journal will publish the results. That conclusion is an error in thinking. There are loads of studies published that did not show statistical significance. The results still are of interest to eye-care professionals: Knowing that treatment A and treatment B are not that different from each other enables doctors to use their judgment to make the best decision for their patients.

The error in thinking that study significance is dependent on statistical significance also can lead to a bad practice known as p-hacking. Basically, the process involves throwing a bunch of mud at the wall and seeing what sticks. Unscrupulous researchers may

- modify the statistical tests, conduct many, or look at multiple variables without adjustments to the alpha level,
- change the inclusion and exclusion criteria to remove data,
- selectively report results (usually only statistically significant results), or
- stop data collection early when a significant result is achieved.

P-hacking, even inadvertently, affects us all. It erodes trust in scientific research, and it leads to false conclusions that can affect future research questions and even patient care.

Using good data diligence when conducting an analysis also involves checking the integrity of the data. When humans are involved, data-entry errors are always possible. Best practice is to check the extreme ends of each variable to catch possible errors.

Here's how such a misstep typically plays out.

Daphne was conducting an investigator-initiated study where one variable should always be a positive number. By checking the range of the data, she was able to spot an entry that had a negative number, reach out to the study coordinator, and have the correct number entered instead. Verifying the variables might not seem like a big deal, but when you are taking the average of 30–50 numbers, huge outliers from data-entry errors can affect the results and ultimately the conclusions. A common error to watch out for with visual acuities is an entry of 0.2 logMAR instead of 0.02 logMAR, or likewise a refraction of ±5.0 D instead of ±0.5 D.

UNDERSTANDING YOUR TOOLS IS CRITICAL TO TRIAL SUCCESS

Tools are great when used properly. Let's look at a specific incident when they were not.

Courtney was a technician at a site tasked with taking visual acuities for an investigator-initiated trial at a private practice. This particular trial used paper worksheets that technicians were supposed to use to calculate the number of letters a participant could read. The instructions were included on the worksheet and, if followed, would end with a final number to be recorded and then used for subsequent analysis.

However, Courtney thought she knew how to use the worksheet and didn't bother to read the instructions. Her final numbers ended up being far fewer than those recorded by other technicians, a discrepancy that was fortunately identified during a review of the data integrity!

The data entries were also able to be corrected with the actual final number of letters read by all the patients from whom Courtney took visual acuities. A disastrous situation was narrowly avoided by good data diligence (such as having worksheets and reviewing the data integrity). Of course, the problem could have been avoided if Courtney had been trained and properly understood the tool that she was using—in this case, the worksheet.

But worksheets are not the only concern in data diligence. Good data diligence means understanding the tools that are used to collect or analyze data. Here is another example.

Jorge had collected data for an investigator-initiated trial in eye care. The data was aggregated in a spreadsheet, and Jorge was tempted by the built-in data-analysis tools within the spreadsheet software. With just a few clicks of the mouse, the software spit out the results of statistical tests, flush with juicy *p* values. However, the wrong statistical tests were used, and the subsequent conclusions drawn were incorrect.

The problem is that the spreadsheet software does not tell you if your statistical test is the correct one for your data or if your data violates the assumptions for that particular test. It just spits out a nice-looking summary of the data. For proper data diligence, Jorge needed to understand the statistical test that was being used **and** whether it was appropriate.

Looking one step further, a lot of researchers have developed tools in eye care to make analysis easier. These products include, but are not limited to, standard graphs for refractive surgery, the Wilcox-Holladay-Wang-Koch statistical software, and mEYEstro software. All are awesome tools, and a big thank-you goes out to all the individuals who develop and make available tools for researchers to use.

My caution, though, is the same as that illustrated by the examples above. You need to understand what these tools do and how to use them before trying them out. Otherwise, you risk using them improperly and drawing the wrong conclusions.

Here's a final example.

Olivia did a study looking at the outcomes of a new intraocular lens. The goal was to publish the results in a medical journal, but the journal required specific figures to be included in any submission. She decided to use a software tool to generate figures for her submission. However, she failed to understand that the data input into the software had to be formatted a certain way for analysis. The details were included in the instructions for using the software, but Olivia ignored them and proceeded anyway. Needless to say, the software did its job and spit out the figure she wanted, but the summary of the data was all wrong since the software excluded all the datapoints that were not formatted correctly. This error was embarrassingly pointed out by a reviewer, and the article was rejected by the medical journal.

Remember that if you are going to use a tool in clinical research, data diligence requires that you understand what it does and how to use it.

MAKE AN IMPACT

- Choose a primary endpoint that will answer your research question.
- Write down two or more secondary endpoints that will provide other insights into your research question.
- List all the critical variables that you will collect during the study.
- With each of the variables in the list you created, write down whether they are continuous, binary, or categorical.
- Consider the statistical tests that are most appropriate for each variable (if applicable)—or reach out to a biostatistician for guidance.

CHAPTER 7:
SHARE THE RESULTS

GETTING THE WORD OUT!

The LENS Share the Results step is about publishing your research in a medical journal and getting on stage at conferences to speak about your outcomes. For your clinical trial to have the greatest impact in eye care, the findings should be disseminated to the greatest number of people possible. A key component of the goal is getting an article about the trial published in a medical journal. You and your colleagues read medical journals to stay on top of the latest research in the field and translate the information into better patient care. By publishing your research in a medical journal, you ensure the findings will be read by other professionals, improving eye care around the world.

Another key component of publishing impact is getting on stage in front of your colleagues at a conference and talking about your trial. A presentation gets you and your research in the spotlight, developing authority and spreading your findings to more people. When people can put a face to an insight, your reputation will improve, and colleagues and sponsors will be more likely to want to collaborate with you in the future.

Sharing your results not only spreads your research to professionals around the world but also drastically increases your impact in eye care as well as frames you and your practice as authority figures in your field. That status will lead to more opportunities for clinical trials, and ultimately, better patient care.

THE SIMPLE METHOD FOR MEDICAL JOURNAL ARTICLE ACCEPTANCE

If you want to create an impact in eye care, then you will need to submit articles for publication in medical journals. Primarily, your article's acceptance by a medical publication will provide validation that your study and results are sound. Any reputable medical journal will invite feedback from your colleagues and experts in the field (peer review) on your particular article. If your reported results are up to snuff, and they advance the field, the article can be published. If not, it will be rejected.

Having your article published in a medical journal means that your study and results are validated and meaningful. In addition, having your study published in a medical journal provides you with recognition. Not only will your colleagues see your name as the author, but potential trial sponsors, grant funders, and collaborators will also take note. So, a double bonus can be obtained from being a published author: (1) improving your standing in the field, and (2) laying groundwork for future partnership opportunities. Finally, when you apply for grant funding, having a list of your published studies is an asset to prove that you can successfully execute a clinical trial and report the results.

Still, you can't simply type up your study and submit it to a journal. Drafting an article that is good enough to be published in a medical journal requires a specialized skill, often referred to as medical writing. The best articles usually tell a good story from start to finish. These are the four key components of a medical journal article:

1. Introduction
2. Methods
3. Results
4. Discussion

The introduction lets the reader know about the current understanding of the research problem, why your study is relevant, and what research question you are trying to answer. Think of an inverted pyramid, and start broadly, getting more and more specific, then finishing with the purpose of your study as the tip of the pyramid at the bottom.

The methods section is by far the easiest section to write. It simply summarizes what you did! It specifies the study design, inclusion and exclusion criteria, relevant surgical or treatment details, study endpoints and how they were collected, and finally, how the data was analyzed. If you created a record in a clinical trial's database—and you should have unless your study is retrospective—then the methods section is a lot like that record but summarized in a more readable format.

The results section is also comparatively easy to write. Here, you are summarizing what you found when you looked at the data. The details include baseline data and all the study endpoints. Whether to include data in the main text, figures, or tables is a matter of taste. However, every field will have conventions, and readers will have expectations that data will be presented a certain way. Therefore, to create a submission that has an impact in eye care, be sure to present the data in similar formats to how they are presented in other studies or recommended by the medical journal you are submitting to.

Finally, the discussion section puts your entire study in context. It is probably the hardest part to write, and it is important to get this section right, as it brings everything together. A poor discussion can lead to rejection, even if the results are groundbreaking. Here is my method to write an effective discussion.

Start with putting your primary endpoint in context, by comparing it to other studies that have already been published, and by linking it to clinical relevance. Work your way down from most important endpoint to least important. Each endpoint can have its own paragraph.

A deep dive is required to properly complete the discussion section and create a lasting impact. You can't spend just a few moments finding some articles that support your conclusions. A proper review of the literature takes hours and hours, and you will need to find all relevant studies to which you can compare your results—especially the ones that disagree with your findings.

In summary, there are just four key sections to master to create powerful publications that are good enough to be featured in medical journals: introduction, methods, results, and discussion.

SURVIVING THE PEER-REVIEW GAUNTLET

When trying to publish a manuscript in a peer-reviewed medical journal, it can really feel like an uphill battle—think Sisyphus, rolling the rock up the hill only for it to be knocked down again. But I promise that if you persevere, you can get through it. Take some comfort in that, for most of the time, it won't be so bad as the example illustrated below.

Ted had submitted the results of an investigator-initiated study to a journal that was less revered but still relevant and read by thousands of eye-care professionals. He received comments back from reviewers about three months later. There were about 30 comments from one particular reviewer, most of which were irrelevant, but he still had to address each point by point, even responding to those comments he disagreed with, stating why. The number was high, but not unusual.

What was unusual was the pushback on five of his responses from this particular reviewer about one month later. He had to again respond to each of those comments, remaining professional, but none were relevant enough to require changes to the text, just for the reviewer's own information. About another month after submitting his responses, he received comments back from the same reviewer! They were addressed with a private note to the editor, but all in all, more than two months of time were lost with the back-and-forth. Ted, having never submitted a manuscript to a medical journal before, was becoming discouraged with each round of revisions. However, instead of giving up, which he felt like doing many times, he persevered and finally got the article accepted! As a published author in a medical journal, he has since been pursued by pharmaceutical companies to conduct further clinical trials.

The point of the scenario is to let you know that ups and downs will come about as you strive to make an impact in eye care—especially when other people are judging your work. But by sticking through the process, you will find success and advance your practice and patient care.

PRESENTING WITH CLARITY AT CONFERENCES

The second big piece of sharing your results is getting on stage and speaking about your research at conferences. Getting your research in front of an appropriate audience allows your colleagues and potential collaborators to put a face to your name—and a face to your research. Professionals want to work with other professionals, so adding the human touch by appearing and interacting at conferences will go a long way to creating a lasting impact in eye care.

One client, Alice, was presenting her research at a conference of her peers. She was given a five-minute time slot to speak about her investigator-initiated trial. The effect that even this small amount of time would have on her life was enormous. Packed in the audience were representatives from some of the biggest pharmaceutical companies in eye care. Some of them were so impressed by her presentation and her research that she was approached right after her talk to discuss future collaboration opportunities with them. Eventually, she started working with these large pharmaceutical companies on other clinical trials, and her career accelerated.

While being center stage at conferences is a great opportunity, the chance can be squandered if you don't do a good job. Through 10-plus years and countless presentations at conferences, I have developed the following tips to help you succeed.

First of all, make a plan! A good presentation tells a good story—and follows a typical structure that covers these points:

1. The background and problem
2. What you did
3. What you found
4. What it means

All parts are crucial but spending too much time in any one area at the cost of another can put your audience to sleep! It's obviously not a great path to recognition.

Second, keep the clutter to a minimum. Avoid the temptation to cram as much information as possible onto each slide, especially if your time slot is limited. Humans have finite attention and will easily turn their brains off—or worse, start glancing at their phones—if you overload them with information. Only include the main points of your research or findings and expand on them when you speak. The same goes for figures and tables. Only include the main data points, and don't put too much information on a single slide, or you will lose the audience—and your opportunity. Make sure the text is large enough even when displayed on a projector to be read from a reasonable distance.

Third, keep the design simple. Sound effects and animations may be encouraged by presentation software, but they distract from the message and can make you look amateurish. The same goes for 3D bar graphs. Don't do it! Before creating a figure or table for a slide, think first if it is something that a medical journal would publish. If the answer is no, then don't include it. If you don't know the answer, then review similar studies in your field that were already published and see how they present data.

Fourth, be sure to grab and maintain attention. When you start your talk, you have only a few seconds to grab attention before minds will wander. Opening with a hook is one way to encourage your audience to pay attention. Find an analogy or other tactic to get their attention immediately.

But how best to keep their attention? Try to refocus your audience's attention periodically during your talk by using cues or having prepared smooth transitions between details as you change slides. Something as simple as "That slide displayed our experimental design, now let me show you what we found" can be an effective cue to refocus your audience on your presentation. You can also cue the audience by summarizing the main idea of each slide before transitioning to the next. For example, "The main takeaway from this slide is to know that treatment A performed better than treatment B initially."

To download a slide template, head on over to https://sengiclinical.com/eyedeatoimpact.

Finally, you likely have heard that the number one rule in real estate is location, location, location. Well, for presentations the rule is practice, practice, practice! If you don't, you can come across as nervous, unprepared, or sloppy, which will reflect badly on you and the research. A good rule of thumb is to run through your presentation at least five times before giving it. Not only will you have practically memorized what you want to say on each slide, ensuring that nothing is missed and your execution will be perfect, but you will also confirm that your talk is on time. A powerful presentation will end almost exactly on time, neither too early nor over the allotted time.

By following the framework above, you will have more effective and powerful presentations, leading to more impact in eye care and gaining the recognition you deserve for all your diligent research work.

CREATING FIGURES AND TABLES THAT MATTER

Writing an article for a medical journal or crafting a slide presentation for a conference talk is a lot like telling a story. If you want to tell a good and powerful story, it helps to have visual aids. Tables and figures fill that need. I have developed a few best practices to make sure these aids add to the overall message and don't detract from it.

To get started, a few overarching principles will determine what constitutes good visual aids. The first might seem obvious, but it does need to be said: Whatever visuals you use, they need to actually be relevant to the overarching story behind your data. For example, a lot of biometry data can be collected for an intraocular lens study, but what's crucial is to include only those data that are relevant to your analysis and study. Too much information can distract the audience from your core message and make your article or talk less effective.

Second, tables and figures need to be clear and simple. They should be able to be understood by a reader without having to search through the main text of your article or by an audience member who may have walked in halfway through your talk. Also make sure that all your tables and figures have the same style, including group labels, font, and color.

Table 5 demonstrates an example of a good table. It can easily be understood without further context because it only contains relevant details as well as relevant *p* values. Moreover, all abbreviations are explained in the footnotes, and all the information is neatly organized.

Table 5: Example of an effective table

Comparison of visual acuity outcomes between treatment groups

Outcome measure	Treatment A (n = 60)	Treatment B (n = 60)	*P* value
Mean change in visual acuity (ETDRS Letters, ± SD)	+12.1 ± 3.8	+9.4 ± 4.2	0.028*
Proportion gaining ≥15 letters (%)	48%	37%	0.15
Proportion losing ≥15 letters (%)	3%	7%	0.18
Central retinal thickness (µm, ± SD)	275 ± 20	285 ± 25	0.08

ETDRS = early treatment diabetic retinopathy study
SD = standard deviation
*Statistically significant at $p < 0.05$

What's a good figure? Figure 2 shows a good example. Both axis titles are clear, as are the numbers and units. It's also simple in that there is only the letter change conveyed, which keeps things plain and avoids clutter. Further, figure 2 contains no unnecessary embellishments, such as 3D effects. (Note that the use of font colors for those who are color-blind also ensures that figures or tables are much more accessible to a variety of audiences. Refer to https://eyesurgeryguide.org/enhancing-visibility-best-colors-for-color-blindness/.)

FIGURE 2

EXAMPLE OF AN EFFECTIVE FIGURE

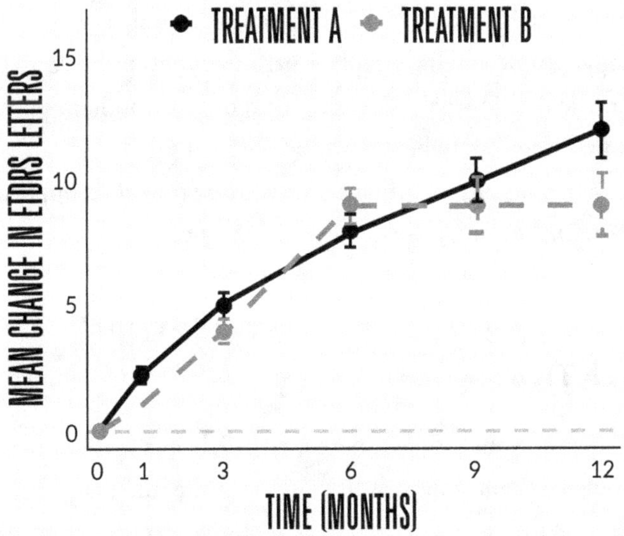

Figure 2: Example of an effective figure

Effective tables and figures should also meet any technical specifications. Medical journals typically specify image resolutions, font sizes, and file formats that are accepted. Likewise, conference presentations should adhere to image quality, font sizes, and file formats as specified, or they should at least work with the presentation platform. Those elements need to be legible to audience members in the back row. Be sure to check out the journal or conference guidelines for more specific directions.

A final note about ethics and copyright—if you are using a table or figure that is not your own original work, then you need to cite your sources! For a conference talk, a good practice is to cite your source on each slide, not at the end of the presentation. For an article in a medical journal, you cannot publish a table or figure that is not your own original work unless it is free of any copyright or you have explicit permission from the copyright holder. Medical journals will ask for proof that you have permission to use the copyrighted work before final publication of your article. Owning the copyright(s) for your own work is important too—original research usually qualifies for a copyright.

WRITING ABSTRACTS THAT CAPTURE ATTENTION

When sharing your results, whether an article in a medical journal or a conference talk, you will also need to make sure that you write an effective abstract. Well-constructed abstracts often are an overlooked piece and can sometimes be the only text that people review before deciding to read your paper or attend your conference talk. Moreover, in competitive conferences, the decision to invite you as a speaker will tend to be based on the abstract. An abstract also provides a first impression of your research. Therefore, to create a lasting impact in eye care, it is crucial to master writing an abstract.

Abstracts, like research articles in medical journals, tend to follow the same structure. That process simplifies the writing task a little bit in that it allows us to go section by section rather than tackling the whole piece. The typical structure is broken in to four sections:

1. Purpose
2. Methods
3. Results
4. Conclusions

The purpose is usually about one sentence and lets the reader know immediately what research question you were trying to answer. The methods section is generally about two to three sentences and lets the reader know what you did. The results are typically two to three sentences and summarize what you found. Finally, the conclusions are one to two sentences that demonstrate how your findings relate to the research question.

In addition to the typical structure, abstracts also have word limits, generally 200–300 words. To have a powerful and effective abstract, you must make sure each word is necessary and adds value to the reader. Writing with vague language is a good way to waste precious words and annoy potential reviewers and readers.

Here is an example of a poor sentence for an abstract: Treatment A affected tear production much more than treatment B.

It not only lacks specifics but leaves out important details.

Here is an improved version: Treatment A increased tear production by 15.4 μL compared to treatment B ($p<0.001$).

Here, we include specific numbers in our comparison and the results of a statistical test.

Because of the word limit, some researchers are tempted to create abstracts that are as close as possible to the limit. That practice can be justified if you have enough valuable things to say, but don't inflate the word count just for the sake of it. Concise writing is expected and is much more effective than an abstract that is longer but has less value per word.

To truly make an impact in eye care, you must make sure that the abstract accurately represents the specifics that will be discussed in your conference talk or journal article. Nothing frustrates a reader or reviewer more than being misled in the abstract. Realize that some of your colleagues will attend your conference talk based on the abstract you have created, and you would do them a disservice by not covering all points mentioned in the abstract in your talk.

Increase your impact and chances of getting accepted or invited by having clarity in your abstract. The best way is by avoiding trade names, acronyms, symbols, and abbreviations where possible. Abbreviations may be useful if the same full meaning would otherwise have to be repeated multiple times, especially to aid in concision. However, I have read so many abstracts where the use of the abbreviation was unnecessary because the word, term, or phrase was only mentioned once! Remember that your abstract may be the only information that is read before someone decides to read your article, attend your talk, or even accept your talk at a conference.

To increase the potential reach of your research—as well as to advance your impact—be sure that you follow proper structure, keep under the word limit, write clearly and concisely, and be consistent with what you will discuss in the publication or on stage.

HOW TO CHOOSE THE RIGHT JOURNAL OR VENUE

By now, you probably understand the importance of sharing your results toward having an impact in eye care. If you have committed to writing a manuscript to submit to a medical journal or to get on stage presenting at a conference of your peers, then you might be wondering which journal or venue is the right one for you!

If your publication has been accepted, the same article cannot be published in more journals. Similarly, most big conferences do not allow encore presentations (because the purpose is to showcase new research). So, take some time and think about your choices before submission! Picking the right medical journal is critical to save time and to reach the greatest number of professionals. Likewise, choosing the best conference to speak at ensures that you are discussing your research with the right audience.

For medical journals, if you are not trying to publish as quickly as possible, then I suggest starting with the top medical journals in your field and speciality.

Why? Because those are the most influential, and generally, more of your colleagues read them than other options. In fact, the top medical journals in your field are likely the journals you receive in the mail on a regular basis! Take a look at recent issues and the author guidelines to determine how well your article will fit into the scope of each journal, then select the most appropriate one. You don't lose anything but time if you submit to a top journal and get rejected. Oftentimes, those journals get a lot more submissions than they can accept—with only about 20%–30% of submitted articles ever getting published.[11,12]

If you receive a rejection, then simply target and resubmit to a lower-impact journal. You can gather a list of them by looking through the articles that you referenced while writing your manuscript. Check out the scope and rank (based on impact factor or another metric) for each journal and decide on a target based on the reviewer feedback from the prior one.

My recommendation would be to select a low-impact journal after rejection from a top-tier journal. The main reason is time! If you wait too long by submitting to other high- or medium-impact journals hoping for acceptance, you run the risk of another researcher

---

11 Suvarna Satish Khadilkar, "Rejection Blues: Why Do Research Papers Get Rejected?," *Journal of Obstetrics and Gynaecology of India* 68, no. 4 (2018): 239–41, https://doi.org/10.1007/s13224-018-1153-1.

12 Rachel Herbert, "Accept Me, Accept Me Not: What Do Journal Acceptance Rates Really Mean?," International Center for the Study of Research (2020), http://dx.doi.org/10.2139/ssrn.3526365.

publishing a similar study before you. That overlap can result in no journal publishing your work since it's no longer unique.

Likewise, when it comes to selecting a conference to submit your abstract to, start with the ones you are already attending on a regular basis! Focus first on the larger, more general conferences in your field. Often, they are the ones that refuse to publish encore presentations. Not only that, but with more overall eye-care professionals attending, your talk will have greater reach and impact. If you receive a rejection from or after presenting at large(r) conferences, you are free to then target smaller regional or subspecialty conferences. Those are often more interactive and fun, but you'll be presenting to fewer colleagues compared to audiences at the big conferences.

For conferences, be sure to pay special attention to their rules. Some conferences—like the American Academy of Ophthalmology (AAO) annual meeting—do not accept presentations based on partially completed studies, so if your study is not complete, then save your time and submit elsewhere. Other conferences have rules against encore presentations. That restriction makes sense because they only want to showcase novel studies for their attendees. An example is the American Society of Cataract and Refractive Surgeons (ASCRS) annual meeting. However, smaller regional meetings are generally more accepting of encore presentations, so you could present at ASCRS first, then elsewhere, but double-check the rules!

One other rule to be aware of is the banning of presentations based on already published studies. For instance, if you submit a manuscript to a medical journal and an abstract to a conference at around the same time, it could be the case that the paper is published **before** your talk at the conference. That situation is one that a conference like the AAO annual meeting wants to avoid. If this happens to you, my suggestion is to talk to the editor at the medical journal and have them delay publication of your article until after the conference. They are usually very understanding, but there is never a guarantee. You could also wait and submit to the journal after the conference too, just to be safe.

RESPONDING CAREFULLY TO FEEDBACK

Nothing is as humbling as being judged by others. Humans are social creatures, and we want others to like us. We want to feel valuable and respected by our peers. Nevertheless, when trying to disseminate your research in a medical journal or on stage at a conference, know and be prepared that you will be judged by others, sometimes very publicly. That truth is often very scary to new researchers and may cause them to hesitate to discuss their research at all. Negative thoughts can make them question their abilities, typically leading to apprehension. These are two common fears:

"What if no journal accepts this paper?"

"What if I get asked a tough question and look foolish on stage?"

Most everyone experiences such worries, but they are often overblown. Sure, some individuals in every facet of life get enjoyment out of trying to embarrass others or will try to make themselves feel better about their own insecurities by lashing out at others. Yet, the vast majority of reviewers and attendees asking questions at conferences genuinely want to make your research better or improve their own understanding.

I encourage you to view feedback as a positive experience, making you stronger and giving your current and future research more impact. In either case, if you want to have powerful publications you will need to know how to respond to feedback. Here are the best practices I have observed in my 15-plus years in research.

FIELDING QUESTIONS AT A CONFERENCE

Let's start with what's often the biggest fear of presenting at conferences, which is getting asked questions! I have found that preparation is key to delivering effective answers to questions and thereby not embarrassing yourself. Prepare by practicing the presentation at least five times before giving it. Through this repetition, you may identify confusing slides and fix them before actually giving the talk. You may also naturally start to think of potential questions that could be asked about the talk and start to formulate responses.

Now, when you are actually on stage it can be quite off-putting to see hands go up, waiting to ask their questions. If you are nervous—everybody gets nervous speaking on stage—remember to breathe. I have found that the best way to begin is to actually listen to the question being asked. Sometimes, you may feel a rush of nervousness and stop listening or start formulating a response in your head to the first part of the question. However, actively listen to the whole question before responding—even in your own head!

If the question has a constructive argument, say so—for example, "Dr. Smith is correct to point out that a limitation of our study is the small sample size."

You can also add explanations, such as "However, we would note that this is interim data, and the final sample will be 100 participants." It is also okay to say that you don't know the answer to the question, but you can offer to discuss the question further with the person at the break or at the end of the conference. In any event, you should be as prepared as possible.

Don't worry about having an answer to every possible question. Realize that you may get asked technical biostatistics questions that are better answered by a biostatistician with whom you work. Being successful in clinical research often means working in teams, so you are not expected to know all the answers. In the case of a particularly hard statistics question, you can politely say that you will have to check with your biostatistician and get back to the questioner at a later time. However, you should be prepared to answer any obvious or typical questions.

KEEPING PERSPECTIVE ON REVIEWER FEEDBACK

Now, let's move on to the harder task of responding to reviewer comments on submitted manuscripts. Written comments from reviewers often sting more than if they were given in person. Part of the reason is that in writing, it is hard to gauge tone, and your brain might interpret a negative, even condescending tone. With written comments, often the reviewers have substantial time to craft a response, so their scrutiny can cut deep.

But don't be discouraged! Remember that all feedback generally makes the research—and you—stronger.

Feedback is usually accompanied by a journal decision, either to reject your manuscript for publication or to reevaluate acceptance after you revise it based on reviewer feedback. Rejection can be really deflating, but remember that it doesn't necessarily mean that the research or writing is terrible. Often the truth is that the study doesn't fit within the scope of the journal, that similar studies were already published on this topic, or that other submissions the journal received scored higher than your submission. If you receive a rejection, take a deep breath, consider their rejection in light of their justification, and resubmit to a different journal.

Having the opportunity to revise your manuscript doesn't guarantee publication to the same journal, however. Moreover, if you do a poor job of responding to comments and editing your paper, you can still be rejected by that journal as well as by another publication. If you follow these upcoming tips, though, you can overcome that obstacle and get your research out there.

A FRAMEWORK FOR RESPONDING

The first thing to remember is that reviewers hold enormous power. They can influence whether a publisher decides to reject or accept your changes and rebuttals. So, be professional in your responses to comments! If you disagree with a recommendation, give good reasons why. You can't just ignore certain comments. You must respond point by point to each comment with either the action you took or the reasons why you disagree with the reviewer. If not, you will annoy the journal editor and are likely to get rejected.

You can make your chances of acceptance higher by creating a stand-alone document that lists each comment. Beneath each comment, politely acknowledge each comment, state how you addressed it and where your clarification can be found, or argue your disagreement with the comment. The key to being effective is to respond objectively, concisely, and completely to each comment.

PUBLISHING MODELS TO CONSIDER—AND AVOID

After getting your article accepted, first congratulate yourself! Really. It is a long road to get there, and you deserve the praise.

Next, you'll have to select a publishing model for your article. The traditional model is one where the journal publishes your article and sends out physical copies to subscribers. The journal makes money by showing ads in the print version as well as by selling subscriptions to universities and individuals. Naturally, the practice works well for the large, established, top-tier medical journals that most of your colleagues read. The advantage to you with this model is that there is no cost. However, any eye-care professional without a subscription to the journal will have a hard time accessing and reading your article, which means there is potentially less impact. Those with significantly less resources will be especially less likely to read your article because full subscriptions or the purchase of individual articles comes with hefty fees.

A relatively new model for publishing is called open access. As the name implies, the access is open, meaning any one can read and download the article free of charge. Open access greatly expands the potential reach of your article. However, because access to the content is free, the journal has to make money elsewhere. The trade-off comes in the form of article-processing charges, which are paid by the authors after article acceptance and before it is made available to the public. Expect to pay a few thousand dollars with the open-access model and be sure to budget for that amount when applying for grants and other funding.

The final publishing model is the one to avoid. I only mention it so that you know to look out for it. Jeffery Beall coined the term "predatory journal" to describe the situation.[13] These companies are more concerned with profit than ethics. Such sources promise rapid review and publication. However, the reality is that there is no peer review, no editorial contributions, no indexing in medical databases, and high fees. The content on these platforms is full of typos, has poor stylistic choices, and looks very unprofessional. It is worse to publish with a predatory journal than to not publish at all! A quick conversation with a colleague or internet search can often be enough to spot and avoid predatory journals.

13 Beall J. Predatory publishers are corrupting open access. Nature. 2012 Sep 13; 489(7415):179. doi: 10.1038/489179a. PMID: 22972258.

I personally believe that making research more accessible will lead to better medical care for everyone. Therefore, I encourage everyone to budget for and to publish via open access. That being said, you should only select this model with journals in your field that have a positive reputation and in which your colleagues also are publishing.

MAKE AN IMPACT

- Identify 1–2 high-impact and 1–2 low-impact journals that align with the scope of your study.
- Review the guidelines for submission to these journals.
- Identify 1–2 conferences where you would like to be on stage speaking about your study.
- Draft the purpose and methods section of an abstract about your study.

PART 3:

PUTTING THE LENS SYSTEM INTO PRACTICE

CHAPTER 8:
CASE STUDIES FROM THE FIELD

CHOOSE YOUR STUDY TYPE

This section will put into practice the information in part 2 and describe three types of studies that you may design.

The easiest study to get started with is a retrospective study. Here, you use already collected patient data to answer a research question. As we will discuss in the following pages, it is the best place for novices to start their journey in investigator-initiated studies.

The prospective type of study, wherein you enroll participants, give an intervention, then follow them for a set number of visits to evaluate the intervention, is one that is probably most often circulated among professionals. A prospective study is more effective than a retrospective study, generally speaking—however, it is also more resource intensive to run.

Somewhere in between a retrospective and prospective study is an ambispective study. With that type of study, patients have already received the intervention, and at your request, they come back into your clinic to collect post-intervention data. An ambispective study is especially useful when retrospective data is not enough to answer your research question.

START WITH A RETROSPECTIVE TRIAL

To get your feet wet in clinical research, the best place to start is a retrospective study. A retrospective trial, as the name implies, looks backward at data that has already been collected. Having a private practice means that you are already sitting on a mountain of data from your patients. However, because patient data will be used, you will need to properly conduct the clinical trial and especially have ethical oversight from an institutional review board or independent ethics committee.

All of the LENS system four-step framework (outlined in part 2) still apply to a retrospective trial. Let's review each of them in more detail.

Launch with Focus

Remember that at this stage you will formulate your research question, choose the type of study, secure funding (if needed), and get approval from an IRB or IEC.

When formulating a research question for a retrospective study, a good place to start is to investigate what already has been published to see if you can identify a gap in the literature. You can start by reading the top-three medical journals in your field to get your creative juices flowing.

While you are coming up with ideas, keep in mind what data you collect and retain as part of your standard of care. Proceeding with a retrospective study to answer a research question is of no use if you don't routinely collect the data to answer it!

Next, determine your study type. The data has already been collected, so you won't be able to have a prospective, randomized, double-masked study. However, consider a couple other study subtypes:

1. Study arms. Will there be a single arm (one group) or multiple arms (multiple groups)?
2. Study sites and investigators. Will you be pulling data only from your patient population, or will you bring in other investigators from your own or other practices?

Next, consider funding. The easiest place to secure funding is from you! You can complete a retrospective trial for as little as a few thousand dollars if you do most of the work yourself. The cost to yourself is the fee you will pay for ethical oversight. Even with an investigator-initiated trial, you can still apply for and use grant funding to pay for the research activities. A good source of outside funding is through the manufacturer of the drug or device in your study design. Favorable results for their product can be a great marketing asset for the company. Reach out to them and pitch your study idea.

Getting IRB or IEC approval is the next step for your retrospective study. Any study using data from humans will need ethical oversight from an IRB or IEC. For a retrospective chart review, the IRB or IEC will likely determine that the research is exempt from ongoing IRB oversight and will also likely grant a waiver of informed consent before you can review patient charts. Without the waiver, each participant will need to consent before you can use their data.

For your application to the IRB or IEC, you will need to prepare essential documents and submit them for approval. Compared to a prospective study, fewer documents are needed in preparation of approval, but a few key ones will be required. Review part 2 for more details on each document:

1. Protocol
2. Curriculum vitae
3. Good clinical practice training
4. IRB-specific forms

The cost for the IRB or IEC is generally between $1,000 and $2,000, although it varies between different providers.

With a retrospective study, there is no requirement to register in a clinical trial registry, such as clinicaltrials.gov, but registration can promote transparency.

Enroll with Confidence

Upon approval, you can mine through your patient chart data and pull out what is relevant to the study based on inclusion and exclusion criteria. If your data is kept primarily in physical charts, then you are going to need to create a spreadsheet and transcribe the key information. If you are short on time, this task is especially good to assign to trusted staff.

Now, if you have electronic health records, aggregating the data may even be easier if you can mass export it. Seek support from your IT staff to complete this function. Data may also be able to be mass exported from diagnostic equipment or surgical suite software. Make sure you don't export personal health information such as names, birth dates, addresses, or email addresses!

Notice the Insights

Once all the data is collected in a spreadsheet and somewhat organized, the fun part begins! The simplest analysis is for a single-arm descriptive study, which involves only doing descriptive statistics: mean, median, standard deviation, percentages, etc.

What you report will depend on the data. Continuous data is usually summarized as mean with standard deviation. Survey data, especially data from nonvalidated surveys, is better summarized using percentages. For example, 47% of participants selected "very satisfied" on the survey at visit 1 compared to 78% at visit 2.

Such simple statistics can generally be completed in most spreadsheet software without the need for statistical software. However, inferential statistics will generally require more robust software. So, unless you are very comfortable with statistics, I recommend hiring a biostatistician for that analysis. Caution is key because a lot of mistakes can be made. Statistical tests also have assumptions that must be met before you can use them. If you blindly use a test without validating the assumptions, the answer you get will be invalid. Remember—garbage in, garbage out.

Once the data analysis is complete, you can breathe a sigh of relief and move onto the next step.

Share the Results

The ultimate aim of most studies is to publish the results! The goal is generally to get published in a peer-reviewed medical journal or to secure speaking engagements on stage at a conference in front of other professionals. Preparing a manuscript for publication or creating slides for a conference talk requires a specialized type of writing known as medical writing. I recommend outsourcing the work to a designated medical writer unless you have the time and skills needed. A well-prepared manuscript may take 40–50 hours of work before being ready for submission to a medical journal!

Both preparing a manuscript and creating a conference talk are pretty similar tasks for a retrospective, prospective, or ambispective study. However, the top medical journal in your field will have a pretty high bar, and retrospective studies are less likely to be published in them. Still, publishing retrospective studies in mid- and low-tier journals is valuable to your standing as a professional in that they can be added to your CV.

The Advantages of a Retrospective Study

Retrospective studies are not inherently better or worse than prospective studies, but they are different.

There is no right or wrong choice, only trade-offs. Here are a few advantages to a retrospective study compared to a prospective study:

1. Simplicity. You might be thinking, "Retrospective studies seem hard to execute." I advise you to keep hesitation to a minimum because if you follow the action steps in this book, you'll find that the process is really quite simple. Moreover, a retrospective study is the easiest way to get started with investigator-initiated trials.
2. Speed. A retrospective study is quick to start because you have already collected the data, and completing the study can also be quick once you have compiled the data into a usable format. Then, all you need is permission and approval from an ethics board or institutional review board, and you'll be off to the races.
3. Cost. If you can or want to do most of the work yourself, the only cost is the IRB fee, which is pretty reasonable compared to the associated expenses of a prospective study. To meet the requirements of a prospective study, you are going to need to pay your staff or a trusted expert to do the extra work involved.

The Disadvantages of a Retrospective Study

On the flip side, here are a couple disadvantages to a retrospective study compared to a prospective study:

1. Less impact than a prospective study. With a retrospective study, the impact is lower than a prospective study,

especially because there's not really a way to randomize. The data is already collected. Even if you had data from a comparator group, the data is less influential than if you had a randomized study of two groups with patients randomized into one or the other group.

2. Limited by data collected. You can also investigate what you have already collected to anticipate its value in your study. If you are missing a certain piece of data or if you used a nonstandardized questionnaire, either one will affect your study. Also, consider that longer and controlled follow-up periods with a prospective study can be more influential than what can be collected retrospectively.

CASE EXAMPLE: RETROSPECTIVE TRIAL

Following is an example of a retrospective investigator-initiated study that I supported with my CRO, Sengi (https://sengiclinical.com/).

The investigator had a large amount of preoperative diagnostic and postoperative data to compare from two devices called biometers. One of the devices was newer, so comparing how well it performed to an already-established device would be relevant to other eye-care professionals. The main purpose of the study was to compare how well these two devices could predict refractive outcomes after cataract surgery and IOL implantation. The secondary purpose was to compare the measurements from each device to see if they provided similar results.

We found that the devices performed similarly well in predicting postoperative outcomes. In addition, minimal differences were observed in the measurements from each device. The study basically revealed that the new device performed as well as the currently available device, so if ophthalmologists used the new device, they could expect similar results for their patients.

The full study is available for free at https://doi.org/10.2147/OPTH.S421504.

Starting with a retrospective study is a great place to step into the realm of clinical research. You will become familiar with the research process and begin to realize the potential benefit to your recognition in the industry and to your practice through clinical research.

A PROSPECTIVE TRIAL IS THE MOST EFFECTIVE

While a retrospective study is the best place to start on your investigator-initiated research journey, prospective studies are the most effective. They are the randomized and double-masked studies that you often see published in the top medical journal of your field. With that type of study, patients receive baseline measurements and an intervention (or more than one), then attend a follow-up visit (or more than one) after the intervention to evaluate its effect. As with a retrospective study, you will need to have ethical oversight from an institutional review board or independent ethics committee and properly conduct the clinical trial. The LENS system will also apply to a prospective trial. Let's review each step and where they differ from a retrospective study in more detail.

Launch with Focus

With a prospective study, you will need to carefully consider a research question, choose the type of study, secure funding (if needed), and get approval from the IRB or IEC.

Compared to the ease of a retrospective study, careful consideration of the research question is needed with a prospective study because prospective studies can take more than one year to collect all the data, plus a few more months to publish. Therefore, you want to select a research question that will be relevant to answer in 12-plus months from the date that you start enrolling. For example, if you know that a new device or drug is coming onto the market in the next 12 months that will make the intervention you want to study obsolete, then don't move forward with your study! Or if the topic has been published already, consider a different question. Publishers, especially medical journals, want to publish novel and relevant studies for their audience of eye-care professionals.

A good place to start thinking about a research topic is to communicate directly with medical device and drug companies. Often, they will provide grant funding for research questions involving their products, but they won't fund the same research idea multiple times. That prerequisite ensures that you are the only one of all related practices doing a clinical trial on that topic.

Also consider your own practice. Did you receive access to a new treatment before your colleagues? If so, it might make a good research topic because you have a competitive edge by being first.

A randomized and double-masked comparative study is the most effective type of prospective studies. Comparative studies (with two or more groups) are effective because the results are put into context (e.g., treatment A is better than treatment B). Randomization ensures that each participant is equally likely to be in either group but is assigned based on random chance. Although not always possible, "masking" participants and study staff to treatment allocations can reduce or eliminate bias from knowing which treatment was assigned. Pooling results from multiple practices can also eliminate investigator- or site-specific biases, such as differential surgical skills and patient demographics.

The drawback with randomized, double-masked comparative studies is the cost in time, resources, and complexity. If applicable, some of that cost can be reduced by having the same participants be assigned to both groups, as it reduces the required number of participants. For example, they could receive treatment A for two weeks, then treatment B for two weeks. Or receive treatment A in one eye and treatment B in the other. Keep in mind, though, that even a single-arm, single-site prospective study can be expensive to conduct. You will have to pay staff, participants, and the IRB or IEC for their time, in addition to the resources allocated from your practice for all the study visits. Outsourced statistical analysis and medical writing will also add to costs.

Because of the relatively higher costs, prospective studies lend themselves well to working with industry partners, such as the manufacturer of the drug or device that you wish to investigate. Being able to show good results with their product can be quite useful for marketing, so some grant funding is often made available. Reach out to industry partners and pitch your study idea.

Remember that any study using data from humans will need ethical oversight from an IRB or IEC. A prospective study requires the same documents as for a retrospective study, plus an informed consent form and any patient-reported outcomes (such as diaries or questionnaires) for review by the IRB. Review part 2 for more details.

For a prospective study, the cost for the IRB or IEC is generally between $3,000 and $5,000, varying among providers.

Remember that you will also need to register the study in a clinical trial registry, such as clinicaltrials.gov.

Enroll with Confidence

Once approved by the IRB or IEC, you can start to recruit study patients. Start with your own patient population. If you need a larger pool of potential participants, then consider partnering with local eye-care professionals for referrals to your study. A strong marketing campaign can also be an asset.

Be sure to keep participants engaged through regular communication from a dedicated study coordinator. In fact, a dedicated study coordinator is the best way to ensure recruitment and retention success. They generally take on responsibility for clinical trial operations and are the point person for participants.

Notice the Insights

With a prospective study, you are going to want a dedicated form to record relevant data from each study visit. Most professionals use paper CRFs because the cost of an electronic data capture system is often prohibitive for an investigator-initiated trial. You can then hand off these CRFs to your biostatistician to deal with, and I do strongly recommend having a dedicated biostatistician for clinical research, especially prospective trials. Their cost is worth it, considering that if the analysis is done improperly then the whole study effort could be a waste. Don't save a penny only to waste a dollar.

Share the Results

Your manuscript and conference talk will be similar regardless of whether your study is retrospective, prospective, or ambispective. However, a prospective study gives you the best chance of success of getting published in top-tier medical journals and thereby having a greater impact. As with publishing a retrospective study, I highly recommend outsourcing to a designated medical writer unless you have the time and the skill, especially if you have the chance to publish in a top-tier medical journal. Editors and reviewers there will have a low tolerance for avoidable mistakes, and a good medical writer will help you navigate this process and give you the best chance to make a high impact.

The Advantages of a Prospective Study

1. High impact. Prospective studies, especially randomized and double-masked studies, have a higher likelihood of

being accepted for publication in top medical journals and for presentation at conferences.

2. Control. You can decide ahead of time what data you want to collect. You are only limited by your imagination and current capabilities.

The Disadvantages of a Prospective Study

On the flip side, you'll find a couple disadvantages to a prospective study compared to a retrospective study:

1. Cost. Prospective studies are generally costlier to run than retrospective or ambispective studies. The increased costs account for paying staff, participants, and the IRB or IEC as well as the time and resources allocated for all the study visits.
2. Time. Prospective studies take the longest to complete. Recruitment, intervention, retention, and follow-up visits take time and typically are spread out over 12 months.

CASE EXAMPLE: PROSPECTIVE STUDY

I have an example of a prospective study that I supported and helped to publish with my CRO, Sengi (https://sengiclinical.com/). The study was a randomized, double-masked, single-surgeon trial that we published in the *Journal of Cataract & Refractive Surgery*, a top-tier medical journal in the field. The comparison involved two, relatively new intraocular lenses (IOLs) to determine how well patients could see objects at various distances (far, intermediate, and near), and the study included a questionnaire.

We found that both IOLs performed well, allowing for patients to see objects clearly at far and intermediate distances, with functional vision for near objects. Interestingly, a difference was revealed in the patient-reported outcomes, with patients noting more visual disturbances with one of the IOLs compared to the other. This study was the first to compare the two IOLs and gave eye-care professionals useful information when suggesting an IOL for their patients.

The full study is available with a subscription from JCRS or through purchase at https://doi.org/10.1097/j.jcrs.0000000000001113.

A prospective study creates the most impact in eye care. If you can navigate the added complexity, cost, and time and successfully complete a prospective study, you will have a better chance of getting accepted to the top conferences and journals.

SAVE TIME AND RESOURCES WITH AN AMBISPECTIVE STUDY

Retrospective studies are a great way to dip your toes into clinical research—prospective studies are the most effective. Ambispective studies, however, sit somewhere in the middle. With an ambispective study, intervention is not a factor (the treatment has already occurred, much like in a retrospective study), and you are bringing in participants to evaluate outcomes after treatment.

Ambispective studies are really good for collecting data that you would not otherwise get with a retrospective study—namely, compiling patient-reported outcomes. If you don't normally give surveys to your patients whom you have already treated, you would need to give them a survey for prospective purposes. You can save time and resources by enrolling patients who already had treatment and have them fill out the survey, rather than meeting the needs of a prospective study where the intervention will be administered and form part of the necessary study visits. Ambispective studies also save time and resources because there is generally only one visit (or e-visit) and no intervention.

As with retrospective and prospective studies, ethical oversight from an institutional review board or independent ethics committee is needed, as is proper conduct of the clinical trial. The four steps of the LENS system will be key to well executing an ambispective study. Let's review each of the steps, and how they differ from retrospective and prospective studies, in more detail.

Launch with Focus

When considering an ambispective study, you generally will be building off retrospective data to include data that you don't normally collect. A great add-on can be a validated questionnaire to gather patient-reported outcomes. Questionnaires are also great because you can provide them in electronic format and thus save patients the burden of having to come into your practice to complete them. Obtaining them electronically saves enormous amounts of time and resources and allows you to complete the study quickly. A prospective study is measured in months from start to finish—an ambispective study is measured in weeks!

To form a good research idea for an ambispective study, think back to the prompts for a retrospective study and see how you might incorporate a questionnaire.

Although ambispective studies are generally more expensive than a retrospective study because of additional IRB or IEC review costs, participant compensation, and staff resources, they are not as expensive as a prospective study. Manufacturers of drugs or devices are a great source of funding—indeed, for all types of studies—because you already have most of the data, which keeps the costs down for sponsors.

IRB or IEC approval is also a little more involved with an ambispective study compared to a retrospective study because the reviewers will need to evaluate and approve the informed consent form and any questionnaires that the study uses. The required documents are the same as for a prospective study, and the cost for the IRB or IEC for an ambispective study is also on par with that of a prospective study. You also will need to register the study in a clinical trial registry, such as clinicaltrials.gov.

Enroll with Confidence

Once you have IRB or IEC approval, you can start to enroll patients. By reviewing chart data of your own patient population, you can generate a list of potential participants and get to work contacting them. The most streamlined approach is to keep the study as digital as you can, which means digital consent forms, video chats, and digital questionnaires. Not only do they help with recruitment by lowering the burden on participants because they don't have to physically come to the office, but electronic formats save staff and clinic resources!

Notice the Insights

Questionnaire data can be tricky to analyze, so I recommend having a dedicated biostatistician help here. Many questionnaires have confusing scoring schemes that can be hard to navigate. Even without complicated scoring, questionnaire data can present difficulties in knowing how to summarize them. Likert-style questions (very dissatisfied, dissatisfied, neutral, satisfied, very satisfied) require special analysis. Considering what is the best way to summarize that data is important. Many investigators are tempted to code the responses as 1 (very dissatisfied) through 5 (very satisfied) and report the average score. However, if you end up with an average score of 4.5, that value doesn't really provide useful information. After all, what would "satisfied-and-a-half" even mean? A better approach would be to summarize the percentages of each response.

Share the Results

With an ambispective study, preparing your conference talk or manuscript is similar to that of a retrospective or prospective study. It is possible to publish in a top medical journal of your field, so don't rule that out. Though less influential than a prospective study, ambispective studies can carry more weight than retrospective studies. For whichever journal you choose to submit to, having a dedicated medical writer will make your life easier because they understand the nuances of technical writing and can navigate all the journal- and conference-specific requirements.

The Advantages of an Ambispective Study

1. Simplicity. A major advantage is the greater simplicity to conduct an ambispective study than with a prospective study, especially so if you use e-consent and electronic questionnaires.
2. Speed. An ambispective study can be a lot quicker to finish that a prospective study—often weeks instead of months!
3. Fewer data limits. With a retrospective study, you are limited to the data that is already collected, but an ambispective study allows you to have another opportunity to evaluate participants and collect more data.

The Disadvantages of an Ambispective Study

On the flip side, a few disadvantages exist in an ambispective study compared to a prospective study.

1. Less impact than a prospective study. An ambispective study will have a lower impact than a prospective study. Since participants have already received treatment, there is no way to randomize to compare one treatment to another even if you had a comparator group.
2. Limited by completed interventions. Your pool of potential participants will be lower compared to a prospective study because you are limited to those patients who have already had an intervention. However, you can examine patient records and get an idea of what the patient pool is ahead of time before committing to the study.

CASE EXAMPLE: AMBISPECTIVE STUDY

Here is a great example of an ambispective study that I supported and helped publish with my CRO, Sengi (https://sengiclinical.com/).

The investigation was a double-arm study performed at a single center. The investigator had been implanting two different presbyopia-correcting intraocular lenses (IOLs) in his patients for almost three years. He was sitting on a mountain of data! Patients who were eligible for the ambispective research were contacted and brought in for one visit. Data was collected to see how well patients could see objects at various distances (far, intermediate, and near), and the study included two different validated questionnaires.

The final total number of participants was 230! We found that both IOLs enabled clear vision at far, intermediate, and near distances, but one performed better to see extremely close objects. We also found that this better performance came at a cost, since the same IOL also had more reports of visual disturbances. All in all, the study was able to be performed more quickly and with fewer resources than a prospective study, and the study still provides useful information for eye-care professionals to consider when discussing IOL choice with their patients.

The full study is available for free at https://doi.org/10.2147/OPTH.S504090.

An ambispective study is a powerful blend of the best parts of retrospective and prospective studies. It has good impact and control because you are able to collect data moving forward but also keeps costs down because the interventions have already occurred.

MAKE AN IMPACT

- Think about a clinical question that you can answer using data that you have already collected to help design an retrospective study.
- Identify one intervention that you would like to design the study around.
- Consider how you could amplify data that you have already collected with patient-reported outcomes.
- Determine which study type you would like to pursue based on your goals and the strengths and weaknesses of each study design.

CHAPTER 9:
EMERGING TRENDS AND OPPORTUNITIES IN INVESTIGATOR-INITIATED TRIALS

A GLIMPSE INTO THE NEAR TERM

In this chapter, we will discuss the future of clinical research, such as the impact of artificial intelligence, decentralized and hybrid clinical trials, adaptive clinical trials, and collaborative research networks. I will share some success stories along the way. Let's get started!

ARTIFICIAL INTELLIGENCE AND ITS IMPACT ON CLINICAL RESEARCH

As I write this section in 2025, artificial intelligence (AI) has really started to affect using investigator-initiated trials to create an impact in eye care—yet perhaps not in the way that most people might think.

Where I think AI tools are going to help medical writers is in completing templates, such as drafting outlines of sections that are expected in a protocol, rather than trying to write those sections. A human should then go through and fill in all the sections and connect the dots.

Similarly, AI tools are a great replacement for search engines. AI can filter through all the ads, SEO, and other unrelated factors and summarize the information in a digestible format. That function saves a lot of time for preliminary research tasks, such as a brief overview of the current understanding of any given topic. But after that initial output, you will have to do a deeper dive with tools such as PubMed.

Another area where I think AI tools are going to help is in the preliminary steps to data analysis by giving answers to specific questions. In that realm, AI can assist a human who understands the data and what needs to happen in order to get the formatting correct or to choose which statistical test to run. In those situations, the human can ask an AI tool for guidance in how to implement what they want to achieve. For a simple spreadsheet, the tool may give you some steps to follow to solve a particular problem. If using a more code-based software (such as R or SAS), then the tool can generally give you some code to use or modify existing code to solve particular problems.

The explosion of AI offers exciting new opportunities for investigator-initiated trials. However, there are critical limitations to be aware of:

1. AI tools can make up information that is not factual (otherwise known as hallucinating). They are also notoriously bad at citing the correct source or even providing a relevant link to where the material could be reviewed.
2. There is significant risk of plagiarism. AI tools are trained by scraping other copyrighted works, and the algorithms are not necessarily programmed to paraphrase or rephrase information to avoid plagiarism.
3. AI tools are inherently always out of date. They are trained by scraping the web and other materials, but that process is not continuous. It is done in batches—perhaps every four to six months a new model comes out, which means that any given model is already months out of date.

These limitations of AI have important implications for investigator-initiated trials, and there are significant risks when using AI tools to begin or to completely draft a protocol or informed consent document for review by an IRB or IEC.

The protocol tells the review board what your study is about, what drug or device you are investigating, and how you plan to answer the research question. Getting these documents aligned with what you actually want for your study is vital. You want to avoid examinations that don't answer the research question, straining your resources and placing an undue burden on patients. Conversely, you shouldn't leave out visits or tests that are crucial for your type of study. The informed consent document should also be truthful and let patients know what the actual treatment will be. If an AI tool gets any of those elements wrong (and you fail to notice), the IRB or IEC will spot the mistake during review. The IRB or IEC will send back the document to you to be corrected and resubmitted for another review by the board, costing time and money.

Consider also manuscript writing. Many journals have strict policies against using text written by AI tools and even images created by these tools. Peer reviewers can't be expected to verify the accuracy of every single piece of text in a given manuscript—that responsibility belongs to the author. Any author who uses AI tools to write their manuscript is shirking their responsibilities to their colleagues, patients, specialty, and science. In addition, if AI is used to conduct a literature review, it will miss all published articles since the model was last updated.

All in all, expect AI to make research more accessible, which is a good thing, but don't forget that AI tools are just tools. A human will still have their place in understanding the overall picture and in overseeing the AI tools to be sure they are used correctly and performing adequately.

THE SHIFTING LANDSCAPE OF INVESTIGATOR-INITIATED TRIALS

Investigator-initiated trials have expanded beyond small, single-site clinical studies. While traditional studies are still immensely valuable, they are not the only way to make an impact in eye care.

The last decade has seen an explosion in computing power, imaging, and infrastructure for health data, which has created new opportunities for research.

The first is conducting retrospective studies using public or registry datasets. These large, de-identified (i.e., stripped of personally identifying information) and highly structured datasets can have millions of patient records—including images—and are a cost-effective way to conduct meaningful research. A few well-known examples are the IRIS Registry (Intelligent Research in Sight), UK Biobank, and All of Us.

Large datasets are also being used to build and validate AI models—for example, diagnostic classification using fundus images, risk stratification from medical record data, or predictive modeling. These data-driven investigator-initiated trials are helping to address key clinical challenges with innovation and automation.

Finally, observational population-based studies don't require an intervention at all. They use data from routine clinical practice to uncover insights to improve patient care. Observational population-based studies can be retrospective or prospective and can answer questions like these:

- Do real-world outcomes differ by age group?
- Are there specific comorbidities that influence disease progression?
- What is the level of patient compliance to treatment or follow-up?

The expanding landscape of trials is exciting but must still be grounded in compliance. The oversight of an IRB or IEC is still necessary. Data that is not fully de-identified, or when linked with another dataset may re-identify patients—therefore, AI, or predictive models, will require additional ethical oversight.

Funding opportunities are evolving as well. Now, many industry partners have grants for projects that develop new AI models, identify unmet needs in patient care, or create new digital tools. On the public side, agencies like the National Institutes of Health (NIH) will support studying novel data science methods to analyze clinical data, create new AI tools, or develop new statistical models.

The types of data-driven studies will benefit greatly from following the LENS system:

1. Launch with Focus. Identify your research question, determine the best dataset to answer it, secure access to the dataset, and get IRB or IEC approval to proceed.
2. Enroll with Confidence. This step involves pulling the right pieces of data from the right datasets to help answer the research question.
3. Notice the Insights. Clean the collected data, analyze it using the right machine-learning or statistical models, and interpret the results for clinical relevance.
4. Share the Results. The expanding landscape of studies is more open, by nature, than traditional investigator-initiated trials, because of the use of public datasets and public funding. As such, it is important to make the results available to the public. One way is by publishing under

the open-access model. Also consider sharing your code and algorithms to maintain transparency and promote collaboration.

CASE EXAMPLE: LARGE DATASETS

Here is a recent case example from the IRIS Registry. Williams et al. looked at loss to follow-up (defined as greater than one year without a clinical encounter) from patients with primary open-angle glaucoma (POAG).[14] They observed that of the approximately 550,000 patients in their study, about half became lost to follow-up and two-thirds never returned for care. What this study demonstrates is the impact that using a large dataset from a registry can have.

As the landscape of investigator-initiated trials evolves to include more data-driven studies, eye-care professionals can lead with innovation and make a lasting impact.

ADVANTAGES OF DECENTRALIZED AND HYBRID CLINICAL TRIALS

If you recall, in chapter 8 we discussed how ambispective studies can leverage technology to eliminate in-person visits, by using e-consent and electronically distributed questionnaires. This development highlights a growing trend in ophthalmology clinical research, known as decentralized trials, whereby all trial-related activities are done outside the clinic (such as at the patient's home).

14 Andrew M. Williams et al., "Loss to Follow Up Among Glaucoma Patients: An IRIS® Registry (Intelligent Research in Sight) Retrospective Cohort Analysis," *Seminars in Ophthalmology* 40, no. 3 (2025): 188–95, https://doi.org/10.1080/08820538.2024.2391826.

There are numerous benefits with this model for your investigator-initiated trials. First, you will have access to a greater pool of potential participants. Having to travel long distances or take time off work can be an enormous burden for participants and cause them to think twice about participating in your investigator-initiated trial. Lowering the barriers allows for greater enrollment and retention. In addition, your time and clinic space are freed up, saving resources. Win-win!

Now that you understand the benefits of decentralized trials, you may be thinking, "How can I incorporate them into my studies?" Here is a list of key activities:

1. Telemedicine. By using secure video, patients could be screened and give consent remotely. Participant follow-up visits and safety monitoring could also be done remotely, depending on the examinations required by your study.
2. E-consent. Documents, like an informed consent form, can now be shared and signed remotely using secure platforms, such as Docusign.
3. ePROs. Questionnaires can be digitized and shared with participants for them to answer remotely at their convenience.
4. Study drug delivery. In certain cases, especially with investigator-initiated trials on already-approved products, study drugs could be dispensed and delivered by a certified third party.
5. Examinations. As technology advances, more and more data collection, such as tonometry, can be done remotely by patients.

Despite recent advances and steps toward making investigator-initiated trials in eye care more decentralized, many study activities can still only be done in the clinic. The list includes a variety of diagnostic equipment such as biometry, topography, fundus photography, optical coherence tomography, and slit lamp examination. Many additional attempts have been made to enable remote visual acuity assessments. However, none are currently sufficient for use in clinical research.

For studies that include examinations that can only be done in the clinic, consider a hybrid approach rather than a fully decentralized trial. A hybrid approach combines both remote and in-person visits to maximize study resources and minimize patient burden. For example, e-consent and screening could be done remotely, with treatment and diagnostics done in the clinic, and patient diaries and surveys done remotely as well.

When considering a decentralized or hybrid model for your next investigator-initiated trial, think about the study population. Ideal participants for these models should have stable medical conditions, be comfortable using technology, and be willing to use more virtual options.

Study staff will also need additional training to make decentralized or hybrid trials a success. First, consider training for the e-consent process, including specifics to the platform that you have chosen. Second, staff should be comfortable with collecting ePROs as well as with monitoring which patients are completing ePROs on time and which need follow-up. Third, technological difficulties will arise, even with patients who consider themselves tech savvy, so staff should be trained in basic troubleshooting. Last, nothing can fully replace an in-clinic visit, so staff should be trained to know when a condition has escalated to the point a participant should be seen on-site.

The IRB or IEC will, of course, need to approve any of the remote features you wish to use in your trial. Many have embraced decentralized and hybrid approaches, but it is worthwhile to check with their customer service before going through the entire application process. To get approval, you will need to show that the remote processes still offer an equivalent level of care (e.g., that IOP measured with an at-home device is as reliable a value as if it were done in the clinic). Also be sure to justify any remote or virtual features. Saving resources is always a good endeavor, but consider patient need first. Does a decentralized or hybrid study allow more geographically diverse patients to participate or decrease the burden to participate overall?

Decentralized and hybrid trials in eye care are an excellent option for investigator-initiated studies. With the right combination of planning, patients, staff, technology, and IRB or IEC buy-in, you can be confident that your next trial will be a success.

MAKE SMARTER DECISIONS WITH ADAPTIVE CLINICAL TRIALS

Did you get the impression that study documents are rigid and unchangeable? Recall from chapter 4 that traditional protocols keep fixed the sample size, treatment arms, endpoints, and analyses.

There is good reason. If sponsors could rewrite protocols on a whim, they would introduce enormous bias into clinical research.

But what if I told you that you could design an investigator-initiated trial protocol that could adapt and change as the study progressed? That capability is the aim of adaptive trial designs, whereby the study protocol contains prespecified rules for how certain elements can be modified based on the data that is being collected. These are examples of changes that can be prespecified:

1. Sample size (larger or smaller)
2. Study arms (eliminate underperforming arms)
3. Inclusion and exclusion criteria (to align with clinical relevance)

Adaptive study designs can be a very useful tool for investigator-initiated trials in eye care. First, the sample size needed for a study can be reestimated partway through the study based on an interim analysis. This review point can allow for early stoppage due to the success or futility of answering the study question, which saves time and resources. Second, study arms can be pruned if performance is lacking (according to an interim analysis), also saving significant time and resources. Finally, many investigator-initiated trials in eye care start with broad inclusion and exclusion criteria. An adaptive design would allow for narrowing of these criteria to focus on a subgroup (identified through an interim analysis) that benefit most from the treatment.

If you want to design an adaptive investigator-initiated study, remember that all potential changes need to be prespecified in the protocol and be able to pass scrutiny by the IRB or IEC. Adaptive trials are more complex to run, so the use of biostatistician is highly recommended as any mid-study changes can affect statistical power and error rates. Performing an interim analysis also introduces the risks of unmasking or bias, so that task should be done by a biostatistician who is independent from the sponsor-investigator.

CASE EXAMPLES: ADAPTIVE STUDY

Lindsey was planning an investigator-initiated study that was going to compare two new IOLs. However, as the IOLs were both new, there was considerable uncertainty about what sample size would allow for meaningful comparisons. Too few and she could fail to spot a true difference in performance—too many and there would be wasted resources and undue burden on patients.

Lindsey decided to use an adaptive design, whereby after 50% enrollment and study completion by participants of the original sample-size estimate, an interim analysis was done, and those results were used to reestimate the sample size. That interval ensured sufficient statistical power, and the study was completed successfully. However, the interim analysis could have also shown that there was very little difference between the groups, and in that case, Lindsey could have stopped the study early, saving resources.

Here is another example. Casey designed an investigator-initiated study with three arms. One arm was the control group, and the other two were variations of the same treatment. A three-arm study takes up a lot of patient time and clinic resources, so Casey decided to use an adaptive design. The plan was to drop one of the variations of the treatment group after 25% of participants were enrolled, based on an interim analysis. The worse performing of the two variations was dropped, and the study was completed with the control and one treatment group.

Adaptive study designs are not just for large clinical trials anymore. With proper planning and support, eye-care professionals can use adaptive designs to improve investigator-initiated trials by reducing wasted time and resources and by improving targeted patient care. The future of clinical research in eye care is flexibility, not rigidity.

UNLOCK THE POWER OF PARTNERSHIPS WITH COLLABORATIVE RESEARCH NETWORKS

An investigator-initiated study doesn't mean that you and your site have to do everything. Enormous opportunities become available when you partner with other sites. Collaborative research networks (CRNs) are structured partnerships between eye-care professionals to conduct clinical studies more efficiently and with greater impact.

Typically, one investigator takes the lead and the role of the sponsor-investigator and brings in partners as subinvestigators. The sponsor-investigator develops a common study protocol plus data collection and management practices, and they obtain overall study approval from the IRB or IEC. Subinvestigators are responsible for getting their site approved by the IRB or IEC and for contributing data from participants.

There are several advantages to using this model if you are the sponsor-investigator. First, access to a larger patient pool enables not only faster recruitment but also the ability to complete studies that require larger sample sizes than your own patient population can support. Second, pooled data from many investigators eliminates site-specific bias (such as a highly acclaimed surgeon) and can increase the generalizability of the results. Third, it saves time and resources for eye-care professionals to form a partnership and conduct one large study than multiple smaller studies. Finally, multicenter studies are implicitly more effective and increase the chances of grant funding and publishing in top-tier medical journals.

Speaking of publishing, being a subinvestigator in a CRN can allow for coauthorship on a peer-reviewed publication or conference presentation. In addition, this contribution can be a great way to dip your toes into the waters of investigator-initiated trials without the added responsibilities of being the sponsor. Keep in mind that you don't have to give up your autonomy to join the partnership.

If you want to start or join a CRN, the best way to begin is to simply start reaching out to colleagues and find those with similar research interests. Once you have nailed down a common research question that you want to answer, be sure to formalize the partnership with an agreement. Typically, it is structured in a clinical trial agreement, a legal contract between the sponsor-investigator and each subinvestigator. Sections should include details about these items:

1. Responsibilities of each party
2. Compensation

3. Data and ownership
4. Intellectual property and publication rights
5. Confidentiality
6. Regulatory compliance

Even with a solid clinical trial agreement, collaborating with others has its challenges. Some can be insufficient recruitment, poor data quality or missing data, and protocol deviations. Effective and frequent communication can reduce or eliminate most issues. I recommend having one point person for all sites to communicate with. A project manager, either internal or from a CRO, would be a great fit for this role.

CASE EXAMPLE: COLLABORATIVE STUDY

Avery wanted to conduct an investigator-initiated trial in eye care, comparing two glaucoma medications. Initial sample-size estimates were far beyond what could be recruited at a single site, so Avery partnered with three other investigators to expand the patient pool. Not only did they achieve 100% enrollment, but by partnering with other eye-care professionals, Avery also was able to complete enrollment ahead of schedule, saving time and resources.

Partnering with colleagues in a CRN can make investigator-initiated trials more efficient, effective, and fun! You don't have to wait to be invited by an industry representative into a multicenter study—you can start your own.

MAKE AN IMPACT

- Pick an area to experiment with AI, such as online searches, documents templates, or code.
- Review your study design and identify any data collection or visits that could be done remotely.
- Consider adaptions (e.g., sample size, study arms, inclusion and exclusion criteria) and determine if your study would benefit from having them prespecified.
- Create a list of colleagues who share your research interests and with whom you would be open to collaborating.

CONCLUSION

Congratulations on completing this book and taking a big step toward creating a lasting impact in eye care.

This book has a lot of information packed within the pages. You learned about the LENS system and its four-step framework for a successful clinical trial: Launch with Focus, Enroll with Confidence, Notice the Insights, Share the Results. All of those concepts are critical to achieving a lasting impact in eye care.

My challenge to you is to act upon what you have read here and not just forget the words and let them slip away. Review the chapters to better absorb the information, if you need to, but do something with the information.

CLINICAL TRIAL TOOLS FOR SUCCESS

I hope by now you are informed about the enormous benefits from undertaking an investigator-initiated trial. I want to share with you not only that knowledge but also the tools for clinical trial success. As a next step, here is what I have for you: resources and templates to aid you in conducting a successful clinical trial. They will help you draft IRB-ready essential documents, recruit patients faster, collect the right data, and boost your chances of getting accepted to speak at a conference or published in a medical journal. These resources are completely free. All you have to do to get them is visit the website below.

Visit www.sengiclinical.com/eyedeatoimpact.

CLINICAL TRIAL SUPPORT

If you are feeling overwhelmed thinking about implementing all the ideas in this book, don't worry! My CRO, Sengi (www.sengiclinical.com/), can help you. Sengi specializes in investigator-initiated trials. We take care of all the paperwork so that you can focus on your patients. We have worked on projects funded by top ophthalmic companies including Alcon, Johnson & Johnson, and Topcon.

Through Sengi's signature method, eye-care professionals receive study start-up support that accelerates timelines, uncovers unique insights through biostatistical analysis, and improves visibility through a focus on conference presentations and peer-reviewed publications.

We are on a mission to simplify clinical research because we believe that more doctors doing good research leads to better medical care for everyone. Partner with us on your study and during our time together, we'll optimize your trial for success. In the first few weeks, we will have completed all start-up activities so that you can hit the ground running with data collection.

Head to www.sengiclinical.com to book a one-on-one with us and see if we are a good fit.

AUTHOR BIO

I knew that I wanted to be involved in medical research since a young age. When I was between 11 and 13 years old, my grandmother and grandfather on my mother's side died of cancer. At the time, my uncle introduced me to the concept of medical research, and I became determined to make a difference.

I became particularly interested in eye research when I was in graduate school, eventually earning my PhD in vision science and biology from the School of Optometry and Vision Science in 2014 at the University of Waterloo in Waterloo, Ontario, Canada.

My PhD research revolved around contact lenses, which brought about my first introduction to clinical research. I completed a study looking at what types of microorganisms can stick to disposable contact lenses—the kind that you use once and throw away. The theory was that they should be relatively clean, but my research found that they were still contaminated.

After finishing my graduate studies, I started a consulting business in which I helped both academics and medical device companies publish their research in related journals and secure positions to speak on stage at conferences. On one of my consulting trips to the U.S., I happened to meet someone who was standing in line to board the same flight. Unbeknownst to me at the time, they would become my mentor and change my business and ultimately my life. Under their guidance, I received specialized training for investigator-initiated trials.

My focus now is supporting eye-care professionals who want to do clinical research by advising, writing, and analyzing data for them. By working directly with investigators, I can do a lot more research and make a bigger impact in eye care because investigators are on the ground floor, directly seeing how different innovations effect patient care. I am honored every day to be a part of that effort by helping them test their hypotheses and ultimately lead to better patient care at a broader scale. My vision for the future is a world where research is more accessible.

ACKNOWLEDGMENTS

This book would not be possible without the knowledge and support of my teachers and mentors over the years. Special thanks to Mom, Dad, Fatima, Lyndon, Jamie, AnnMarie, and Rick.

www.ingramcontent.com/pod-product-compliance
Lightning Source LLC
LaVergne TN
LVHW011512200926
848484LV00001B/22